15683135

X

MW00716537

Leonard A. Jason
Joseph R. Ferrari
Margaret I. Davis
Bradley D. Olson
Editors

Creating Communities
for Addiction Recovery:
The Oxford House Model

Creating Communities for Addiction Recovery: The Oxford House Model has been co-published simultaneously as *Journal of Prevention & Intervention in the Community*, Volume 31, Numbers 1/2 2006.

Pre-publication
REVIEWS,
COMMENTARIES,
EVALUATIONS . . .

"THIS INFORMATIVE BOOK is at once a systematic evaluation of an important intervention for addiction and a vivid illustration of the value of strengths-based community psychology research. Along the way, the authors show how the process of community research and the amount of knowledge it uncovers are enhanced by a respectful, dynamic relationship between academic scientists and community-based organizations."

Keith Humphreys, PhD
Associate Professor of Psychiatry,
Stanford University

"THIS IS AN EXCEPTIONAL, INSPIRING EXAMPLE OF COLLABORATIVE ACTION RESEARCH: A university team of community psychologists and an innovative community-based organization, working as partners in each step of the research. Their exemplary work HOLDS BOTH SCHOLARLY AND PRACTICAL VALUE FOR COMMUNITY PSYCHOLOGY AND FOR SUBSTANCE ABUSE RECOVERY. This research has implications at multiple ecological levels, involving personal recovery within a supportive residential community; organizational functioning of an innovative community setting; the role of physical environmental factors in recovery; understanding how recovery can be promoted among diverse populations; and social policy on substance abuse recovery."

James H. Dalton, PhD
Professor of Psychology
Bloomsburg University of Pennsylvania

"AN IMPORTANT BOOK that will give communities and states greater confidence in supporting the creation of more Oxford Houses, which are critically needed especially now when there are fewer long-term altrernatives for those with serious addictions. It is important that the larger addiction community and gatekeepers learn about Oxford Houses as they provide a critical element for those who are working to maintain their sobriety."

Greg Meissen, PhD
Director and Professor of Psychology,
Self-Help Network:
Center for Community Support
and Research,
Wichita State University

The Haworth Press, Inc.

Creating Communities for Addiction Recovery: The Oxford House Model

Creating Communities for Addiction Recovery: The Oxford House Model has been co-published simultaneously as *Journal of Prevention & Intervention in the Community*, Volume 31, Numbers 1/2 2006.

Journal of Prevention & Intervention in the Community is the successor title to *Prevention in Human Services,* which changed title after Vol. 12, No. 2 1995. *Journal of Prevention & Intervention in the Community,* under its new title, began with Volume 13, No. 1/2 1996.

Creating Communities for Addiction Recovery: The Oxford House Model, edited by Leonard A. Jason, PhD, Joseph R. Ferrari, PhD, Margaret I. Davis, PhD, and Bradley D. Olson, PhD (Vol. 31, No. 1/2, 2006). *"This informative book is at once a systematic evaluation of an important intervention for addiction and a vivid illustration of the value of strengths-based community psychology research. Along the way, the authors show how the process of community research and the amount of knowledge it uncovers are enhanced by a respectful, dynamic relationship between academic scientists and community-based organizations." (Keith Humphreys, PhD, Associate Professor of Psychiatry, Stanford University)*

Psychological, Political, and Cultural Meanings of Home, edited by Mechthild Hart, PhD, and Miriam Ben-Yoseph, PhD (Vol. 30, No. 1/2, 2005). *Examines the meaning of home as a psychologically, spiritually, politically, or physically challenging experience.*

Technology Applications in Prevention, edited by Steven Godin, PhD, MPH, CHES (Vol. 29, No. 1/2, 2005). *Examines new prevention options made possible by today's cutting-edge technology.*

Six Community Psychologists Tell Their Stories: History, Contexts, and Narrative, edited by James G. Kelly, PhD, and Anna V. Song, MA (Vol. 28, No. 1/2, 2004). *"Should be required reading for any student aspiring to become a community psychologist as well as for practicing community psychologists interested in being provided unparalleled insights into the personal stories of many of the leading figures within our field. This book provides readers with an inside look at the reasons why a second generation of community psychologists entered this field, and also provides a rare glimpse of the excitement and passion that occured at some of the most important and dynamic community training settings over the past 40 years." (Leonard A. Jason, PhD, Professor of Psychology and Director, Center for Community Research, DePaul University)*

Understanding Ecological Programming: Merging Theory, Research, and Practice, edited by Susan Scherffius Jakes, PhD, and Craig C. Brookins, PhD (Vol. 27, No. 2, 2004). *Examines the background, concept, components, and benefits of using ecological programming in intervention/prevention program designs.*

Leadership and Organization for Community Prevention and Intervention in Venezuela, edited by Maritza Montero, PhD (Vol. 27, No. 1, 2004). *Shows how (and why) participatory communities come into being, what they can accomplish, and how to help their leaders develop the skills they need to be most effective.*

Empowerment and Participatory Evaluation of Community Interventions: Multiple Benefits, edited by Yolanda Suarez-Balcazar, PhD, and Gary W. Harper, PhD, MPH (Vol. 26, No. 2, 2003). *"Useful . . . . Draws together diverse chapters that uncover the how and why of empowerment and participatory evaluation while offering exemplary case studies showing the challenges and successes of this community value-based evaluation model." (Anne E. Brodsky, PhD, Associate Professor of Psychology, University of Maryland Baltimore County)*

Traumatic Stress and Its Aftermath: Cultural, Community, and Professional Contexts, edited by Sandra S. Lee, PhD (Vol. 26, No. 1, 2003). *Explores risk and protective factors for traumatic stress, emphasizing the impact of cumulative/multiple trauma in a variety of populations, including therapists themselves.*

Culture, Peers, and Delinquency, edited by Clifford O'Donnell, PhD (Vol. 25, No. 2, 2003). *"Timely . . . . of value to both students and professionals. . . . Demonstrates how peers can serve as a pathway to delinquency from a multiethnic perspective. The discussion of ethnic, racial, and gender differences challenges the field to reconsider assessment, treatment, and preventative approaches." (Donald Meichenbaum, PhD, Distinguished Professor Emeritus, University of Waterloo, Ontario, Canada; Research Director, The Melissa Institute for Violence Prevention and the Treatment of Victims of Violence, Miami, Florida)*

Prevention and Intervention Practice in Post-Apartheid South Africa, edited by Vijé Franchi, PhD, and Norman Duncan, PhD, consulting editor (Vol. 25, No.1, 2003). *"Highlights the way in which preventive and curative interventions serve–or do not serve–the ideals of equality, empowerment, and participation. . . . Revolutionizes our way of thinking about and teaching socio-pedagogical action in the context of exclusion." (Dr. Altay A. Manço, Scientific Director, Institute of Research, Training, and Action on Migrations, Belgium)*

Community Interventions to Create Change in Children, edited by Lorna H. London, PhD (Vol. 24, No. 2, 2002). *"Illustrates creative approaches to prevention and intervention with at-risk youth . . . . Describes multiple methods to consider in the design, implementation, and evaluation of programs." (Susan D. McMahon, PhD, Assistant Professor, Department of Psychology, DePaul University)*

Preventing Youth Access to Tobacco, edited by Leonard A. Jason, PhD, and Steven B. Pokorny, PhD (Vol. 24, No. 1, 2002). *"Explores cutting-edge issues in youth access research methodology. . . . Provides a thorough review of the tobacco control literature and detailed analysis of the methodological issues presented by community interventions to increase the effectiveness of tobacco control. . . . Challenges widespread assumptions about the dynamics of youth access programs and the requirements for long-term success." (John A. Gardiner, PhD, LLB, Consultant to the 2000 Surgeon General's Report* Reducing Youth Access to Tobacco *and to the National Cancer Institute's evaluation of the ASSIST program)*

The Transition from Welfare to Work: Processes, Challenges, and Outcomes, edited by Sharon Telleen, PhD, and Judith V. Sayad (Vol. 23, No. 1/2, 2002). *A comprehensive examination of the welfare-to-work initiatives surrounding the major reform of United States welfare legislation in 1996.*

Prevention Issues for Women's Health in the New Millennium, edited by Wendee M. Wechsberg, PhD (Vol. 22, No. 2, 2001). *"Helpful to service providers as well as researchers . . . A useful ancillary textbook for courses addressing women's health issues. Covers a wide range of health issues affecting women." (Sherry Deren, PhD, Director, Center for Drug Use and HIV Research, National Drug Research Institute, New York City)*

Workplace Safety: Individual Differences in Behavior, edited by Alice F. Stuhlmacher, PhD, and Douglas F. Cellar, PhD (Vol. 22, No. 1, 2001). Workplace Safety: Individual Differences in Behavior *examines safety behavior and outlines practical interventions to help increase safety awareness. Individual differences are relevant to a variety of settings, including the workplace, public spaces, and motor vehicles. This book takes a look at ways of defining and measuring safety as well as a variety of individual differences like gender, job knowledge, conscientiousness, self-efficacy, risk avoidance, and stress tolerance that are important in creating safety interventions and improving the selection and training of employees.* Workplace Safety *takes an incisive look at these issues with a unique focus on the way individual differences in people impact safety behavior in the real world.*

People with Disabilities: Empowerment and Community Action, edited by Christopher B. Keys, PhD, and Peter W. Dowrick, PhD (Vol. 21, No. 2, 2001). *"Timely and useful . . . provides valuable lessons and guidance for everyone involved in the disability movement. This book is a must-read for researchers and practitioners interested in disability rights issues!" (Karen M. Ward, EdD, Director, Center for Human Development; Associate Professor, University of Alaska, Anchorage)*

Family Systems/Family Therapy: Applications for Clinical Practice, edited by Joan D. Atwood, PhD (Vol. 21, No. 1, 2001). *Examines family therapy issues in the context of the larger systems of health, law, and education and suggests ways family therapists can effectively use an intersystems approach.*

Creating Communities for Addiction Recovery: The Oxford House Model

Leonard A. Jason
Joseph R. Ferrari
Margaret I. Davis
Bradley D. Olson
Editors

Creating Communities for Addiction Recovery: The Oxford House Model has been co-published simultaneously as *Journal of Prevention & Intervention in the Community*, Volume 31, Numbers 1/2 2006.

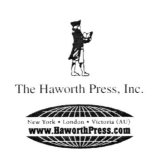

The Haworth Press, Inc.

New York • London • Victoria (AU)
www.HaworthPress.com

Creating Communities for Addiction Recovery: The Oxford House Model has been co-published simultaneously as *Journal of Prevention & Intervention in the Community*™, Volume 31, Numbers 1/2 2006.

The Haworth Press, Inc., 10 Alice Street, Binghamton, NY 13904-1580 USA

Cover design by Kerry E. Mack

Cover illustration, "Oxford House," by Bradley D. Olson

Library of Congress Cataloging-in-Publication Data

Creating Communities for Addiction Recovery: The Oxford House Model / Leonard A. Jason. . . [et al.], editors.
      p.cm
      "Co-published simultaneously as Journal of prevention & intervention in the community, volume 31, numbers 1/2 2006."
      Includes bibliographical references and index.
      ISBN10:   0-7890-2929-4 (hard cover : alk.paper)
      ISBN13:   978-0-7890-2929-4 (hard cover : alk.paper)
      ISBN10:   0-7890-2930-8 (soft cover : alk.paper)
      ISBN13:   978-0-7890-2930-0 (soft cover : alk.paper)
      1. Oxford House, Inc. 2. Substance abuse–Treatment–United States. 3. Recovering addicts–Services for–United States. 4. Recovering alcoholics–Services for–United States. 5. Halfway houses–Unirted States. 6. Self-help groups–United States. I. Jason, Leonard. II. Journal of prevention & intervention in the community.
HV4999.2.O93 2006
362.29'185–dc22

                                                  2005003562

Indexing, Abstracting & Website/Internet Coverage

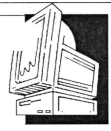

This section provides you with a list of major indexing & abstracting services and other tools for bibliographic access. That is to say, each service began covering this periodical during the year noted in the right column. Most Websites which are listed below have indicated that they will either post, disseminate, compile, archive, cite or alert their own Website users with research-based content from this work. (This list is as current as the copyright date of this publication.)

Abstracting, Website/Indexing Coverage . . . . Year When Coverage Began

- *Behavioral Medicine Abstracts* **1996**
- *Business Source Corporate: coverage of nearly 3,350 quality*
  magazines and journals; designed to meet the diverse
  information needs of corporations; EBSCO Publishing
  <http://www.epnet.com/corporate/bsourcecorp.asp> **2003**
- *CINAHL (Cumulative Index to Nursing & Allied Health*
  Literature), in print, EBSCO, and SilverPlatter, DataStar,
  and PaperChase. (Support materials include Subject
  Heading List, Database Search Guide, and instructional
  video). <http://www.cinahl.com> **2003**
- *EBSCOhost Electronic Journals Service (EJS)*
  <http://ejournals.ebsco.com> **2001**
- *Educational Research Abstracts (ERA) (online database)*
  <http://www.tandf.co.uk/era>. **2002**
- *EMBASE.com (The Power of EMBASE + MEDLINE*
  Combined) <http://www.embase.com>. . . . . *
- *EMBASE/Excerpta Medica Secondary Publishing Division.*
  Included in newsletters, review journals, major reference works,
  magazines & abstract journals <http://www.elsevier.nl> **1996**
- *e-psyche, LLC <http://www.e-psyche.net>* **2001**
- *Excerpta Medica . . . See EMBASE* . . . . *
- *Family & Society Studies Worldwide <http://www.nisc.com>* **1996**

(continued)

(continued)

　　* **Exact start date to come.**

Special Bibliographic Notes related to special journal issues (separates) and indexing/abstracting:

- indexing/abstracting services in this list will also cover material in any "separate" that is co-published simultaneously with Haworth's special thematic journal issue or DocuSerial. Indexing/abstracting usually covers material at the article/chapter level.
- monographic co-editions are intended for either non-subscribers or libraries which intend to purchase a second copy for their circulating collections.
- monographic co-editions are reported to all jobbers/wholesalers/approval plans. The source journal is listed as the "series" to assist the prevention of duplicate purchasing in the same manner utilized for books-in-series.
- to facilitate user/access services all indexing/abstracting services are encouraged to utilize the co-indexing entry note indicated at the bottom of the first page of each article/chapter/contribution.
- this is intended to assist a library user of any reference tool (whether print, electronic, online, or CD-ROM) to locate the monographic version if the library has purchased this version but not a subscription to the source journal.
- individual articles/chapters in any Haworth publication are also available through the Haworth Document Delivery Service (HDDS).

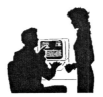

ABOUT THE EDITORS

Leonard A. Jason, PhD, is Professor of Psychology at DePaul University, in Chicago, where he heads the Center for Community Research. He has published 384 articles and 65 chapters on recovery homes for the prevention of alcohol, tobacco, and drug abuse; preventive school-based interventions; media interventions; chronic fatigue syndrome; and program evaluation. He has been on the Editorial Boards of seven peer-reviewed psychology journals, and he has edited or written seventeen books. He has served on review committees of the National Institute of Drug Abuse and the National Institute of Mental Health, and has received more than $16 million in federal grants to support his research. He is former President of the Division of Community Psychology of the American Psychological Association and a past Editor of *The Community Psychologist*. He has received three media awards from the American Psychological Association, and he is frequently asked to comment on policy issues for the media.

Joseph R. Ferrari, PhD, is Professor of Psychology at DePaul University, Chicago, Illinois. Along with Dr. Jason, he has studied the benefit of Oxford House for men and women in recovery since 1993. The author of over 120 scholarly publications and 350 conference presentations, Dr. Ferrari is an international speaker and scholar on applied psychology topics, including community volunteerism, caregiver stress and satisfaction, child safety in retail stores, and psychological sense of community, eldercare, and behavioral applications to social problems. Dr. Ferrari is Editor of the *Journal of Prevention & Intervention in the Community* (The Haworth Press: NY), Director of the Masters of General Psychology and former Director of the Doctorate in Community Psychology, both at DePaul. He also is a motivational speaker for businesses and non-profit organizations.

Margaret I. Davis, PhD, is Assistant Professor of Psychology at Dickinson College, Carlisle, Pennsylvania. She received her PhD in Clinical-Community Psychology from DePaul University and for four years served as Sr. Project Director on a NIDA-funded grant studying Oxford House self-run recovery homes for substance abuse at DePaul University's Center for Community Research. The professional manuscripts she has published primarily focus on the issues of collaborative research, and social support and women in the realm of substance abuse and recovery. Dr. Davis has also served as a program evaluator and consultant to the Chicago Mayor's Office for People with Disabilities. Her interests include the evaluation of substance abuse treatment programs, the study of substance use and recovery issues for women, the interplay of social and personal resources, and the development of self-advocacy skills and empowerment of youth with disabilities.

Bradley D. Olson, PhD, is an addictions researcher at DePaul University and an advocate supporting a greater national emphasis on healthcare-based approaches toward alcohol and substance abuse problems. He has published numerous research articles, many on consumer-run recovery homes, and has provided congressional testimony, once on the relationship between substance abuse and crime and again on the feasibility of faith-based initiatives. He is chair of U.S. Congressman Danny K. Davis' drugs and substance abuse advisory committee and chairperson of CATCH (Citizens Activated to Change Healthcare). CATCH, in conjuction with Congressman Davis' office, those in recovery, treatment providers, and many others obtained roughly 118,000 signatures from registered voters to get a treatment-on-demand initiative on the Cook County ballot in Illinois. On November 2nd, 2004, 1.2 million people (76%) voted in support of the referendum.

Creating Communities for Addiction Recovery: The Oxford House Model

CONTENTS

Preface

The papers comprising this special volume are the result of research conducted in the context of a 13-year collaborative action research partnership between DePaul University and Oxford House, Inc., a community-based organization (CBO). Founded in 1975, Oxford House is a system of self-supported, democratically operated homes that offer residents recovering from substance abuse problems a mutual-help setting to develop long-term abstinence skills (Jason, Davis, Ferrari, & Bishop, 2001). The ultimate goal of this university-CBO partnership was the on-going assessment of this innovative model for recovery via multiple methods of data collection. In keeping with principles of collaboration, community members and other relevant parties were consistently engaged to inform and actively shape these endeavors to our mutual benefit.

Several of the chapters herein (e.g., Brown, Davis, Jason & Ferrari; Ponitz, Olson, Jason, Davis, & Ferrari; and Flynn, Alvarez, Jason, Olson, Ferrari, & Davis) utilized data collected as part of two large NIH-funded studies that are currently underway, with Leonard Jason as Principal Investigator and Joseph Ferrari as Co-Principal Investigator. The first project was funded by NIAAA as a five year, randomized outcome study within the state of Illinois (Bradley Olson, Project Director). In this study, 150 individuals who agreed to participate were randomly assigned to either a "usual aftercare" condition or Oxford House upon discharge from a traditional in-patient treatment program. Individuals in both conditions were interviewed upon entry to the study and then interviewed every 6 months for two years. The second project was funded by NIDA using an accelerated longitudinal design to examine the relation between social support for abstinence, the development of self-efficacy, and successful abstention from substance use in a national sample of Oxford House residents (Margaret Davis, Project Director). In the NIDA study, approximately 900 individuals completed

[Haworth co-indexing entry note]: "Preface." Jason, Leonard A. et al. Co-published simultaneously in *Journal of Prevention & Intervention in the Community* (The Haworth Press, Inc.) Vol. 31, No.1/2, 2006, pp. xix-xx; and: *Creating Communities for Addiction Recovery: The Oxford House Model* (ed: Jason et al.) The Haworth Press, Inc., 2006, pp. xvii-xviii. Single or multiple copies of this article are available for a fee from The Haworth Document Delivery Service [1-800-HAWORTH, 9:00 a.m. - 5:00 p.m. (EST). E-mail address: docdelivery@haworthpress.com].

surveys every four months for 16 months. Additionally, a minority supplement was obtained to explore cultural diversity within Oxford House, particularly among Latino populations (Josefina Alvarez, Project Director).

Throughout the years of the partnership, the DePaul team has also conducted a number of smaller-scale studies of Oxford House and the research process (e.g., see Jason, Davis, Olson, Ferrari, & Alvarez, in this volume). These studies have focused on both local and national residents (e.g., in this volume, see d'Arlach, Olson, Jason, & Ferrari), involved both qualitative and quantitative data regarding inner-, inter-, and intrapersonal variables and processes (e.g., see Davis, Dziekan, Horin, Jason, Ferrari, & Olson; and Kim, Davis, Jason, & Ferrari, in this collection), as well as contextual characteristics and policy implications (e.g., see Braciszewski, Olson, Jason, & Ferrari; Ferrari, Jason, Blake, Davis, & Olson; Ferrari, Jason, Sasser, Davis, & Olson; and Olson, Viola, Jason, Davis, Ferrari, & Rabin-Belyaev, in this volume), in order to explore experiences of recovery and Oxford House settings in greater depth. The results of several of these studies are also highlighted.

Leonard A. Jason
Joseph R. Ferrari
Margaret I. Davis
Bradley D. Olson
Editors

PART 1:
THE COLLABORATIVE
PROCESS

Chapter 1:
Cultivating and Maintaining Effective Action Research Partnerships:
The DePaul and Oxford House Collaborative

Margaret I. Davis

Dickinson College

Bradley D. Olson
Leonard A. Jason
Josefina Alvarez
Joseph R. Ferrari

DePaul University

SUMMARY. In this paper, we review the result of research conducted in the context of a 13-year collaborative partnership between DePaul

Address correspondence to: Margaret I. Davis, PhD, Dickinson College, P.O. Box 1773, Carlisle, PA 17013-2896 (E-mail: davismar@dickinson.edu).

The authors would like to thank Paul Molloy and the men and women of Oxford House who shared their stories, insights, and experiences in this collaborative process and devoted time and interest to participate in each of the research projects. The authors also thank the numerous students and volunteers who assisted in data collection and analysis for these projects.

Funding for this manuscript was made possible by grants from the National Institute on Alcohol Abuse and Alcoholism (Grant #AA12218) and the National Institute on Drug Abuse (Grant #DA13231).

[Haworth co-indexing entry note]: "Chapter 1: Cultivating and Maintaining Effective Action Research Partnerships: The DePaul and Oxford House Collaborative." Davis, Margaret I. et al. Co-published simultaneously in *Journal of Prevention & Intervention in the Community* (The Haworth Press, Inc.) Vol. 31, No. 1/2, 2006, pp. 3-12; and: *Creating Communities for Addiction Recovery: The Oxford House Model* (ed: Jason et al.) The Haworth Press, Inc., 2006, pp. 3-12. Single or multiple copies of this article are available for a fee from The Haworth Document Delivery Service [1-800-HAWORTH, 9:00 a.m. - 5:00 p.m. (EST). E-mail address: docdelivery@haworthpress.com].

University and a community-based, self-run, residential substance abuse recovery program called *Oxford House*. This collaborative effort high-lights several examples of the research and action activities fostering a positive alliance that benefited both the research team and the Oxford House community. It also proposed practical guidelines for developing effective action research collaboratives that may be helpful to others who desire to cultivate and maintain similar mutually beneficial partner-ships; including such processes as the development of trust, respecting the personal experiences of the community members and group, com-mitment to serving the community, validating findings with organiza-tion members, and accountability. *[Article copies available for a fee from The Haworth Document Delivery Service: 1-800-HAWORTH. E-mail address: <docdelivery@haworthpress.com> Website: <http://www.HaworthPress.com> © 2006 by The Haworth Press, Inc. All rights reserved.]*

KEYWORDS. Oxford House, participatory research, action research

Community psychology advocates that in order to better understand and intervene within communities, researchers need to venture out of their traditional universities and interact with individuals in the social framework of their settings (Dalton, Elias, & Wandersman, 2001; Kingry-Westergaard & Kelly, 1990). Researchers need not only seek to become familiar with the complex contexts and processes that comprise community functioning, but also to seek community input, community effort, and community ownership in these endeavors (Jason, 1997). One strategy adopted by community psychologists is to work in partnership with CBOs, within their fabric and structure, shifting from the role of detached observer and expert to collaborator and facilitator (see Rappaport & Seidman, 2000; Sandler, 2001). According to the field of community psychology, many of the most complex and intransigent so-cial and community problems can be transformed by the recognition, appreciation, and utilization of the assets and inner resources that al-ready exist within those social settings (Jason). Working in collabora-tion provides an opportunity to identify and build upon these resources, and allows for more accurate and sensitive evaluation of the commu-nity-based organization and its programs, which in turn may be utilized to improve the delivery and efficacy of services (Gomez & Goldstein, 1996; Ostrom, Lerner, & Freel, 1995).

Despite the great benefits to be gained from cultivating and maintain-ing collaborative research partnerships, initiating and preserving such efforts create unique challenges that must be addressed in order to sustain a mutually beneficial alliance throughout the research process. The 13-year relationship between DePaul University and Oxford House illustrates the dynamic process of collaborative work highlighting practical issues that may be encountered when collaborating with a CBO, and how the unconventional paradigm of inquiry and action is most appropriate and effective when working with such organizations and groups.

The history of the partnership between the DePaul University research team and Oxford House and the adoption and evolution of this collaborative action-research agenda is detailed elsewhere (see Jason, Davis, Ferrari, & Bishop, 2001; and Suarez-Balcazar, Davis, Ferrari, Nyden, Olson, Alvarez et al., 2004). However, several instances are summarized below that capture the mutually-beneficial nature of the collaborative. Although these examples primarily highlight action endeavors, in research efforts, the DePaul team also collaborated with Oxford House members in all aspects of the development, design, and implementation of projects. Oxford House maintains a meaningful leadership role throughout the research process, and members of the Oxford House community fully supported the efforts of the DePaul group by becoming a part of our research team and serving as data collectors and field researchers (see Jason, Davis, Olson, Ferrari, & Alvarez, in the collection, for a study on the impact of their participation in this process). Additionally, many Oxford House residents have accessed university resources and taken advantage of the services we offer (e.g., consultation regarding house issues, suggestions on grants and other funding sources, etc.).

From initial contact onward, the DePaul research team engaged the Oxford House community as active participants and endeavored to maintain the alliance. The University team not only strived to cultivate collaborative and cooperative relationships with Oxford House, but also became committed to active involvement in the process of creating change. Some examples of endeavors that the research team has undertaken in collaboration with Oxford House include the involvement in the establishment of the first Men's, first Women's, and first Women with Children's Oxford Houses in Illinois, as well as historical and ongoing involvement in activities that support the national growth of Oxford House.

For example, in 1992, Oxford House, Inc. sent a representative to Chicago in order to begin the establishment of Oxford Houses in the area, but funding complications occurred at Illinois Department of Alcohol and Substance Abuse (DASA) that left the representative without necessary housing and financial support. The University team offered to provide the representative with free accommodations–first at the home of one of the members of the research team and then at a DePaul University residence. The staff also provided the representative with office space, a telephone, and other resources to facilitate his efforts. Because of this joint effort, the first Illinois Oxford House home was successfully established in Chicago. The home was located near the University and graciously named the *DePaul House*.

Additionally, DePaul was involved with the establishment of Oxford Houses for women and women with children in Illinois. In 1994, Jason and Ferrari obtained small grants to support the funding of a female recruiter to establish two women's houses in the Chicago area. The DePaul group joined with Oxford House to form a committee to create the job description and conduct interviews with potential candidates for the recruitment position. Once hired, Oxford House arranged for the new recruiter to visit women with children's homes in Missouri, where she stayed in order to learn more about the founding and working of successful homes. The DePaul team provided the recruiter with an office, phone, training, and supervision; offered expertise regarding group and community dynamics; and worked closely with her throughout the process-providing advice and support during stressful times. Through this joint effort, the recruiter succeeded in opening two Chicago-based Women's Oxford Houses in 1995, including a Women and Children's House (McSherry, 1995). The following year, as the end of the grant was approaching, the DePaul team also assisted the recruiter in obtaining a position with Illinois DASA to continue her work on behalf of women in recovery.

As evidenced in these examples, the intent has been to foster a positive alliance that will ultimately benefit both the researchers, who are interested in investigating the dynamics and supporting the growth and development of the Oxford House model, and the recovery community, which appreciates the expertise and support that the University team can provide.

Guidelines for Effective Action Research Collaboratives

Based on this research, we develop the action research collaborative (ARC) model to describe critical points that may serve as practical guidelines for those who desire to cultivate and maintain similar collaborative partnerships (see Table 1).

1. *Cultivate Trust.* At the foundation of the collaborative endeavor was the *cultivation of trust* between members of the University and the community (Fetterman, 1996). Since initial contact with

Oxford House, the DePaul team has consistently worked to build mutual trust and dispel misconceptions. The development of this trust was without doubt aided by the inclusion of OH residents and recovering individuals on the research team, who were able to more easily access and establish rapport with Oxford Houses based on their shared understanding of addiction and recovery processes and, in general, facilitated a greater openness to dialogue (McCrady & Miller, 1993).

2. *Open Lines of Communication.* The research team also found it paramount to initiate and maintain *open lines of communication* among all relevant and interested parties. Ongoing open and honest communication on procedures, general issues, and problems that may arise during the research process insures collaboration and reduces mistrust among parties (Harper & Salina, 2000).

3. *Look for Opportunities to Promote Social Justice and Change.* Consistent with the ideals of community psychology, we maintain that researchers undertaking collaborative enterprises also must *look for opportunities to promote social justice and change* that best serve the community's interest. The DePaul team's efforts to date have included utilization of media and dissemination of information to influence agency and government decision-making. Additionally, there have been numerous and innovative means to actively work toward creating change on multiple and broad levels (see Jason, 1991; and in this volume, Braciszewski, Olson, Jason, & Ferrari; and Olson, Viola, Jason, Davis, Ferrari, & Rabin-Belyaev for examples).

4. *Look to Mobilize and Utilize Existing Resources.* Collaborative enterprises can also be enhanced when researchers *look to mobilize and utilize existing resources* (Nyden, Figert, Shibley, & Burrows, 1997). These resources include those possessed by the university, the community, and other agencies. For example, Jason knew state officials concerned with substance abuse prevention and intervention from previous research projects and drew upon these relationships as the DePaul team worked as advocates for Oxford House in Illinois. Members of the Oxford House community have likewise contributed many valuable resources to the partnership over the years, including their participation, support and insight, suggestions on methodology and measures, and feedback on findings.

5. *Accommodate Diverse Agendas.* Additionally, collaborative partnerships often require the *accommodation of diverse agendas.*
   The research team's ongoing dialogue with Oxford House and
   other participating agencies provided the opportunity to learn the
   varied needs of diverse parties and reconcile agendas through
   communication and compromise.

6. *Bring Respect.* It is also critical that researchers *bring respect* to
   the collaboration process. The research team members need to respect the dignity, opinions, ideology, expertise, and needs of the
   community and the individuals who comprise it (e.g., see Ponitz,
   Olson, Jason, Davis, & Ferrari, in this volume). Further, as advocates and researchers working within a contextualist-ecological
   framework (Kingry-Westergaard & Kelly, 1990), we must respect the processes that occur within the community. Throughout
   the years of our collaborative partnership, we have created and revised our agenda, studies, methods, and measures based upon a
   deep appreciation for community members' insights and input
   (Davis, Jason, Ferrari, Olson, & Alvarez, in this volume).

7. *Operationalize and Validate Results Within Context.* Consistently,
   we have capitalized on valuable opportunities to *operationalize and
   validate results within context,* which may be one of the greatest assets of conducting research within the fabric and structure of a
   community. For, while laboratory-based research may control for
   certain confounding variables, it is often at the cost of compromis-
   ing other types of validity that limit the applicability of findings to
   real-world settings (see Cook & Campbell, 1979; Cronbach, 1975;
   for discussion of these issues). Conducting collaborative research
   within environments where social processes actually occur provides unique opportunities to assess and rule out threats to internal
   validity (thereby increasing confidence in causal inferences), to
   more accurately define operational constructs and clarify related
   contingency limitations to generality, and to explicate possible restrictions to external validity (Cook & Campbell; Tebes, 2000).
   Collaborative research provides a rich context for critically understanding phenomena of interest. Thus, the DePaul team has con-
   tinuously sought the involvement of and feedback from members
   of the community to clarify concepts and to validate our results.

8. *Reflect Critically on One's Roles, Values, and Attitudes.* We have
   found that it is also important to *reflect critically on one's roles,*

values, and attitudes. Unlike the traditional research paradigm where researcher-participant roles are clearly defined and it is recommended that personal values be suspended for the sake of objectivity, the boundaries within a collaborative approach become less clear and values are held to be an integral part of the community research endeavor (Shadish, 1990). Throughout our research and action endeavors it has been important for team members to reflect upon their personal and professional values, explore the implications of adopting multiple roles, and openly discuss issues that might impact decisions.

9. *Appreciate the Dynamics of Role Evolution.* Likewise, we have come to *appreciate the dynamics of role evolution.* Different participants in the collaborative relationship have different skills that will be brought to the research process. Over time, individual's roles and relationships change. For example, during the course of our projects, research assistants and Oxford House residents have become employees, consultants, graduate students, and Project Directors; and both community and research team members have moved on to become employees of other agencies (e.g., see Jason et al., in this volume). The DePaul-Oxford House relationship has also experienced qualitative changes over the years as both organizations have continued to grow, and our bonds have been strengthened as we have engaged in this long-term mutually-supportive partnership.

10. *Take a Strengths-Based Approach.* Additionally, it is most consistent with our values, the values of community psychology, and the values of the community, to *take a strengths-based approach* in our endeavors. While much of the substance abuse and addiction literature focuses on relapse, enabling, denial, and a host of pathological personal and interpersonal traits often attributed to recovering individuals, our focus has been on the strengths of this community (e.g., in this volume, see Davis, Dziekan, Horin, Jason, Ferrari, & Olson). Oxford House is a strengths-based model that, like 12-step programs, emphasizes the mutual sharing of experience, strength, and hope. In our research, we attempt to capture and explore the strengths of this program–studying the ability of members to heal and grow in this mutual-support approach toward recovery. For example, we examine concepts such as social support (e.g., see Kim, Davis, Jason, & Ferrari, in this volume), sense of

community (e.g., see d'Arlach et al.), self-liberation, helping behaviors, conflict resolution skills, hope, and self-efficacy among House members, as well as individual, interpersonal, and community resources that may facilitate recovery (e.g., in this volume, see Brown, Davis, Jason, & Ferrari; Ferrari, Jason, Blake, Davis, & Olson; and Flynn, Alvarez, Jason, Olson, Ferrari, & Davis).

11. *Exeunt Gracefully.* Last, but not least, is the necessity to "*exeunt gracefully.*" Even when separation from a community-based organization, such as Oxford House, is not encroaching, one must be sensitive to the fact that in order to eventually accomplish this, one must consider issues related to exiting the community long before it is imminent. Indeed, it is essential to consider these issues from the commencement of the partnership and throughout the collaborative process. As such, to exit gracefully ultimately requires that one begins gracefully and remains graceful throughout. This end can also be served by inviting ongoing and open communication and maintaining cognizance of both the community's expectations and how the research endeavor can and will impact the community. Because a primary responsibility of community psychologists is to improve communities in a lasting way, in working with the Oxford House, we have actively attempted to impact their organization and community in ways that will serve to support and empower.

TABLE 1. Guidelines for Developing and Maintaining Effective Action Research Collaboratives (ARCs)

Cultivate trust

Open lines of communication

Look for opportunities to promote social justice and change

Look to mobilize and utilize existing resources

Accommodate diverse agendas

Bring respect

Operationalize and validate results within context

Reflect critically on one's roles, values, and attitudes

Appreciate the dynamics of role evolution

Take a strengths-based approach

Exeunt gracefully

REFERENCES

Braciszewski, J. M., Olson, B. D., Jason, L. A., & Ferrari, J. R. (2006). The influence of policy on the differential expansion of male and female self-run recovery settings. *Journal of Prevention & Intervention in the Community, 31* (1/2), 51-62.

Brown, J. T., Davis, M. I., Jason, L. J., & Ferrari, J. R. (2006). Stress and coping: The roles of ethnicity and gender in substance abuse recovery. *Journal of Prevention & Intervention in the Community, 31* (1/2), 75-84.

Cook, T. D., & Campbell, D. T. (1979). *Quasi-experimentation: Design and analysis issues for field settings.* Boston: Houghton Mifflin.

Cronbach, L. J. (1975). Beyond the two disciplines of scientific psychology. *American Psychologist, 30*(2), 116-127.

Dalton, J. H., Elias, M. J., & Wandersman, A. (2001). *Community psychology: Linking individuals and communities.* Belmont, CA: Wadsworth/Thomson Learning, Inc.

Davis, M. I., Dziekan, M. M., Horin, E. V., Jason, L. A., Ferrari, J. R., & Olson, B. D. (2006). Women leadership in Oxford House: Examining their strengths and challenges. *Journal of Prevention & Intervention in the Community, 31* (1/2), 133-143.

Davis, M. I., Jason, L.A., Ferrari, J. R., Olson, B. D., & Alvarez, J. (in press). A collaborative action approach to researching substance abuse recovery. *American Journal of Drug and Alcohol Abuse.*

Ferrari, J. R., Jason, L. A., Blake, R., Davis, M. I., & Olson, B. D. (2006). "This is my neighborhood": Comparing United States and Australian Oxford House neighborhoods. *Journal of Prevention & Intervention in the Community, 31* (1/2), 41-49.

Fetterman, D. M. (1996). Empowerment evaluation: An introduction to theory and practice. In D. M. Fetterman, S. J. Kaftarian, & A. Wandersman (Eds.), *Empowerment evaluation: Knowledge and tools for self-assessment and accountability.* Thousand Oaks, CA: Sage Publications.

Flynn, A. M., Alvarez, J., Jason, L. A., Olson, B. D., Ferrari, J. R., & Davis, M. I. (2006). African American Oxford House residents: Sources of abstinent social networks. *Journal of Prevention & Intervention in the Community, 31* (1/2), 111-119.

Gomez, C. A., & Goldstein, E. (1996). The HIV prevention evaluation initiative: A model for collaborative and empowerment evaluation. In D. M. Fetterman, S. J. Kaftarian, & A. Wandersman (Eds.), *Empowerment evaluation: Knowledge and tools for self-assessment and accountability.* Thousand Oaks, CA: Sage Publications.

Harper, G. W., & Salina, D. D. (2000). Building collaborative partnerships to improve community-based HIV prevention research: The university-CBO collaborative partnership model. *Journal of Prevention & Intervention in the Community, 19,* 1-20.

Jason, L. A. (1991). Participating in social change: A fundamental value for our discipline. *American Journal of Community Psychology, 19,* 1-16.

Jason, L. A. (1997). *Community Building, Values for a Sustainable Future.* Westport, CT: Praeger Publishers.

Jason, L. A., Davis, M. I., Ferrari, J. R., & Bishop, P. D. (2001). Oxford House: A review of research and implications for substance abuse recovery and community research. *Journal of Drug Education, 31,* 1-27.

Jason, L. A., Davis, M. I., Olson, B. D., Ferrari, J. R., & Alvarez, J. (2006) Attitudes of community members as a function of participatory research with Oxford Houses. *Journal of Prevention & Intervention in the Community, 31* (1/2), 13-24.

Kim, K. L., Davis, M. I., Jason, L. A., & Ferrari, J. R. (2006). Structural social support: Impact on adult substance use and recovery attempts. *Journal of Prevention & Intervention in the Community, 31* (1/2), 85-94.

Kingry-Westergaard, C., & Kelly, J. G. (1990). A contextualist epistemology for ecological research. In P. Tolan, C. Keys, F. Chertok & L. Jason (Eds.), *Researching community psychology: Issues of theory and methods.* (pp. 23-31). Washington, DC: American Psychological Association.

McCrady, B. S., & Miller, W. R. (1993). *Research on Alcoholics Anonymous: Opportunities and alternatives.* New Brunswick, NJ: Rutgers Center on Alcohol Studies.

McSherry, M. (1995, January 2). Struggling down road to recovery: DePaul helps moms stay straight. *The Daily Southern,* pp. 1.

Nyden, P., Figert, A., Shibley, M., & Burrows, D. (1997). *Building community: Social science in action.* Thousand Oaks, CA: Sage Publications.

Olson, B. D., Viola, J. J., Jason, L. A., Davis, M. I., Ferrari, J. R., & Rabin-Belyaev, O. (2006). Economic costs of Oxford House compared to inpatient treatment and incarceration: A preliminary report. *Journal of Prevention & Intervention in the Community,* 31 (1/2), 63-72.

Ostrom, C. W., Lerner, R. M., & Freel, M. A. (1995). Building the capacity of youth and families through university-community collaborations: The Development-In-Context Evaluation (DICE) model. *Journal of Adolescent Research, 10,* 427-448.

Ponitz, J. E., Olson, B. D., Jason, L. A., Davis, M. I., & Ferrari, J. R. (2006). Medical care of individuals residing in substance abuse recovery homes: An analysis of need and utilization. *Journal of Prevention & Intervention in the Community, 31* (1/2), 95-110.

Rappaport, J., & Seidman, E. (Eds.). (2000). *Handbook of community psychology.* New York: Kluwer/Plenum Publishers.

Sandler, I. (2001). Quality and ecology of adversity as common mechanisms of risk and resilience. *American Journal of Community Psychology, 29,* 19-61.

Shadish, Jr., W. R. (1990). Defining excellence criteria in community research. In P. Tolan, C. Keys, F. Chertok & L. Jason (Eds.), *Researching community psychology: Issues of theory and methods.* (pp. 9-20). Washington, DC: American Psychological Association.

Suarez-Balcazar, Y., Davis, M., Ferrari, J., Nyden, P., Olson, B., Alvarez, J., Molloy, P., & Toro, P. (2004). Fostering university-community partnerships: A framework and an exemplar. In L. A. Jason, C. B. Keys, Y. Suarez-Balcazar, R. R. Taylor, M. I. Davis, J. Durlak, & D. Isenberg (Eds.), *Participatory community research: Theories and methods in action.* Washington, D.C.: American Psychological Association.

Tebes, J. K. (2000). External validity and scientific psychology. *American Psychologist, 55*(12), 1508-1509.

Chapter 2:
Attitudes of Community Members
as a Function of Participatory Research
with Oxford Houses

Leonard A. Jason

DePaul University

Margaret I. Davis

Dickinson College

Bradley D. Olson
Joseph R. Ferrari
Josefina Alvarez

DePaul University

SUMMARY. Citizen participation in research may include involvement in generating original ideas, planning appropriate designs, collecting data, and helping to implement interventions. Unfortunately, little is

---

Address correspondence to: Leonard A. Jason, PhD, Center for Community Research, DePaul University, 990 West Fullerton Avenue, Chicago, IL 60614.

The authors would like to thank Paul Molloy and the men and women of Oxford House who participated in each of the research projects for sharing their insights and experiences in this collaborative process.

The research described in this paper was supported by grants from the National Institutes of Health (NIAAA, Grant #AA12218; and NIDA, Grant #DA13231).

[Haworth co-indexing entry note]: "Chapter 2: Attitudes of Community Members as a Function of Participatory Research with Oxford Houses." Jason, Leonard A. et al. Co-published simultaneously in *Journal of Prevention & Intervention in the Community* (The Haworth Press, Inc.) Vol. 31, No.1/2, 2006, pp. 13-24; and: *Creating Communities for Addiction Recovery: The Oxford House Model* (ed: Jason et al.) The Haworth Press, Inc., 2006, pp. 13-24. Single or multiple copies of this article are available for a fee from The Haworth Document Delivery Service [1-800-HAWORTH, 9:00 a.m. - 5:00 p.m. (EST). E-mail address: docdelivery@ haworthpress. com].

known about the attitudes of the community members who participate in such research processes. In the present exploratory study, a team of community members (4 men, 3 women; age > 30 years old) who were employed as investigator research associates to evaluate an innovative substance abuse recovery home, were asked for their perspectives about their involvement in the research effort. Findings indicated that these community members felt their participation was a positive experience. Moreover, while their understanding and sense of participation in the research process increased, their identification and affiliation with their support organization was not reduced. Results imply that there is a need to better understand how citizen members of community organizations are affected by their involvement in the research process. *[Article copies available for a fee from The Haworth Document Delivery Service: 1-800-HAWORTH. E-mail address: <docdelivery@haworthpress.com> Website: <http://www.HaworthPress.com> © 2006 by The Haworth Press, Inc. All rights reserved.]*

KEYWORDS. Collaboration, citizen participation, participatory action research

Participatory research has been described as an "attitude" that prioritizes the needs and interests of the people in the research context and invites full participation in decisions about design, implementation, and the utilization of results (Chataway, 2001). Kelly (1990) considers the collaborative endeavor a *discovery process*, in which the different parties share their individual constructions of their contexts, learn about events and processes that help define their understanding of the contexts, and work together to define the intervention activity. Integrating research methodology with community initiatives focused on improving the quality of life of citizens has been found to nurture participants' personal growth, increased self-esteem, a sense of belonging to a larger community, and empowerment over social ills (Ferrari & Jason, 1996).

When working collaboratively with citizens, researchers need to address several issues (Jason & Glenwick, 2002). First, it is important to decide if it is appropriate to involve citizens in the research. This decision may be influenced by (a) the rules or requirements of the community or the funding source, (b) the type and scale of the research and its relevance to the community, or (c) the researcher's resources and expectations about the effects of citizen involvement (Wandersman, Chavis, & Stuckly, 1983). Second, if the research lends itself to citizen involvement, then it is important to determine the best level of involvement. Wandersman et al. described five levels of participation, ranging from noninvolvement (i.e., citizens are not informed of the results of the research) to complete involvement (i.e., citizens play a primary role in the project). Regardless of the level of participation, investigators have infrequently assessed the experience of the community members in the research effort (Jason et al., 2004). It is likely that involving community members in the research process impacts on these individuals, but it is unclear whether such involvement cultivates more self-competence, a critical understanding of the research process, and skills and resources for further community and political action (Keiffer, 1984).

Citizen participation might enhance ways of understanding a variety of community problems (Jason et al., 2004), such as the social problems of drug and alcohol addiction. Consider, for instance, the high rates of recidivism following treatment for a variety of physical and mental disorders. After treatment for substance abuse from hospital-based treatment programs, therapeutic communities, or recovery homes, many clients return to former high-risk environments or stressful family situations. Returning to these settings without a network of people to support abstinence may increase chances of a relapse (Montgomery, Miller, & Tonigan, 1993). As a consequence, substance abuse recidivism following treatment is high for both men and women. In addition, under modern managed care, private and public sector inpatient substance abuse facilities have reduced their services dramatically. There is currently a rising interest in citizen participation and self-help groups because they offer an empowerment orientation and may be more cost-effective than more professionally directed treatments.

Oxford House, founded in 1975, illustrates a community-based approach toward substance abuse abstinence (Jason et al., 1997). Unlike traditional hospital care where trained professionals are necessary, or therapeutic communities where residents have a maximum length of stay, Oxford House offers a community where residents can live without the involvement of professional treatment staff and where there are no time restrictions on length of stay. Because there is no maximum stay, residents may have a greater opportunity to develop a sense of competence toward maintaining abstinence. Similar to 12-step programs, members of an Oxford House receive abstinence support from peers; however, unlike AA or NA there is no single, set course for recovery that all members must follow. Rather, residents of Oxford House are free to decide personally whether to seek psychological or substance abuse treatment by professionals or 12-step programs. In short, Oxford

House offers residents the freedom to decide whether to seek and choose which (if any) treatment they desire while receiving constant support and guidance within an abstinent communal setting.

Settings such as Oxford House that are self-governing, and require minimal costs because the residents pay for their own expenses, including housing and food, are particularly promising given the current cost-conscious environment and need for successful cost-effective approaches to treat drug abuse. Additionally, the recovery home experience of communal living may offer residents several specific benefits. Recovering substance abusers living in these settings report a strong sense of bonding with similar others who share common abstinence goals (Jason et al., 1997). Receiving abstinence support, guidance, and information from recovery home members committed to the goal of long-term sobriety and non-drug use can enable substance abusers to reduce the probability of a relapse. This experience can provide residents with peers who can model effective coping skills, be resources for information on how to maintain abstinence, and act as advocates for sobriety. Further, because grassroots movements have helped expand the number of Houses to over 1,000 within 48 states, this alternative to traditional residential programs has become more widely accessible.

In an effort to evaluate this network of Oxford Houses, several research studies were mounted and members of the Oxford House organization were actively involved in the research projects. The present brief study was conducted in order to explore the impact of research participation on the citizens who were members of the Oxford House community and involved in the research effort. The following domains were assessed: amount of dialogue and communications, the ways decisions were made, their influence regarding research and implementation issues, their investment and level of trust in the research project, their knowledge about research methods, their feeling as being part of the research team, as well as their identification with the research team and the Oxford House organization.

METHOD

Description of Studies and Oxford House Members

Members of the Oxford House organization participated in two large-scale community-based studies. The first project, funded by the National Institute on Alcoholism and Alcohol Abuse (NIAAA), was a randomized outcome study within the state of Illinois. In that study, 150 individuals finishing a traditional in-patient treatment program were randomly assigned to either a "usual aftercare" condition or Oxford House. The participants assigned to the Oxford House condition were introduced to an Illinois Oxford House, where the current residents interviewed and determined whether to accept the individual into their home. Individuals in both conditions were interviewed upon entry to the study and then every 6 months for two years.

On this study, there were two Oxford House members who served as recruiters. One recruiter was a male and the other recruiter was a female (age > 30 years old; one was African-American and one was Caucasian). A recruiter was a full-time employee who recruited individuals from the treatment centers, tracked and interviewed participants, entered interview data, and attended weekly research meetings.

The second project, funded by the National Institute on Drug Abuse (NIDA), used an accelerated longitudinal design to examine the relation between social support for abstinence, the development of self-efficacy, and successful abstention from substance use in a national sample of Oxford House residents. In that study, approximately 900 individuals were recruited from various geographic locations where the majority of Oxford Houses tend to cluster. The participants completed surveys every four months for a 16 month period.

At the time of this study, there were three full-time and two part-time Oxford House recruiters who worked on this project. Two full-time recruiters were female and one full-time and two part-time recruiters were male. Two were African-American and four were Caucasian (age > 30 years old). Similar to the recruiters in the NIAAA study, these citizen researchers were involved in both recruiting and interviewing participants over the various waves of the study.

Dependent Variables

After approximately 1.5 years of participation on the project, the seven Oxford House citizen recruiters were asked to fill out a "Process Questionnaire." The recruiters were informed that this information would be helpful to the researchers for understanding their feelings concerning their participation in the research project. Recruiters were asked to indicate how they felt using a 9-point scale when they first joined the research team as well as at the current time. Ratings were conducted on the following items: *amount of dialogue and communications between the Oxford House recruiters and the DePaul University researchers* (from no dialogue to considerable), *method of decision making* (from not democratic to very democratic), *influence regarding research is-*

sues (from none to considerable), *influence regarding implementation of the project* (from none to considerable), *investment in the research project* (from none to considerable), *level of trust in the research project* (from none to considerable), *degree of personal identification with DePaul University or Oxford House* (1 = identification with DePaul, 5 = identification with both settings, 9 = identification with Oxford House), *knowledge about research methods* (from none to considerable), and *feeling part of the research team* (from none to considerable).

RESULTS

Recalled initial and post ratings from the seven Oxford House community representatives are in Figure 1. Given the small sample size, the Wilcoxon Signed ranks test was employed. Significant pre-post

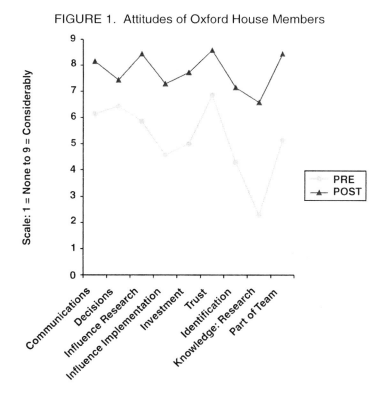

FIGURE 1. Attitudes of Oxford House Members

changes were found for 6 of the 9 dimensions: amount of dialogue and communications ($Ms = 6.1$ to 8.1, $z = -1.93$, $p = .05$), influence regarding research issues ($Ms = 5.9$ to 8.4, $z = -2.25$, $p < .05$), influence regarding implementing the project ($Ms = 4.6$ to 7.3, $z = -2.23$, $p < .05$), investment in the research project ($Ms = 5.0$ to 7.7, $z = -1.90$, $p < .05$), knowledge about research methods ($Ms = 2.9$ to 6.6, $z = -2.38$, $p < .05$), and feeling part of the team ($Ms = 4.3$ to 8.4, $z = -2.23$, $p < .05$).

Directional positive changes also occurred regarding the way decisions were made and their trust in the research project. On the item involving their degree of personal identification with DePaul University and Oxford House (with 1 = DePaul University, 5 = both, and 9 = Oxford House), the mean ratings changed from 4.3 to 7.1. Although this change was not significant, the direction of the change suggests that participation in the research effort actually served to increase rather than reduce their identification with the Oxford House self-help organization.

These Oxford House members also provided us written comments about their experience on the research team, which serve to elucidate the impact of their involvement in the research process.

> I would say that the best part of working on the NIDA project was working with such a diverse group of individuals, both on staff, and of course the participants. I definitely improved on my communication skills, as well as salesmanship. There were many times that I was required to go in and sell the idea to a group of men or women to participate in this study. Different approaches for different people. I was also grateful to learn more about my self-discipline, and at times, lack there of. The job gave me the opportunity to share what worked and what didn't, take advice and direction from others, as well as give support to my co-workers. The group of us, I would say, definitely formed into a family, similar to that of Oxford House. I am thankful for the two years we shared.

> I think the first and a very important change as a result of participating in the project is that it has given me focus in what I want to do professionally in my life. Before this job, I was swimming around in jobs that were not careers and not knowing what direction I wanted to go in (job wise and education wise). This job opened my eyes to a new area of study/work and made me realize that I wanted to continue work in this or a related area. I had never had a job where I felt such meaning or purpose. I am truly thankful

to DePaul for this–I'm not sure you realize what a significant impact this opportunity has had in my life. Secondly and also related, as being part of a research team, I felt that my ideas and experience were really important and valued in the shaping of this study. I think that this was the first time that I had really felt this way in a job. It gave me self confidence and made me realize that I had something, a lot to offer. At the same time, being part of such an open-minded, nurturing research team allowed me the opportunity to really open my mind and learn a lot of new things and different ways to look at things. Lastly, this experience has given me more insight into people/substance abusers. I had plenty of experience looking at substance abuse as a recovering addict in recovery and doing service work but it was almost as if I got to see it from the other side of the coin, the research aspect. How do people, other people/researchers view substance abuse? What makes up people? There were so many different measures that looked at different aspects of people–I think of people and what experiences make up people differently now. This experience has also enhanced my ability to relate to people and form connections with people I have just met. Also, it has enhanced my ability to get across my ideas to people who I have just met. I thought I had a couple sentences to write and then I started writing and couldn't stop!! This is a testimony to the wonderful experience I have had with DePaul and the large amount of change this job has had in my life!

Working as a research recruiter for DePaul has been rewarding in so many ways to say the least. At the very beginning I felt valued and accepted as an individual by my superiors and all the members of the team. It has been wonderful to work with such understanding and supportive people. I have expanded my knowledge of Psychology from the courses I took in college, which were very basic to include Community and Social Psychology, because of the broad knowledge base of our team and their fields of study. I remain teachable, and learn more with every team meeting as I hope I bring my team members a better understanding of what addiction and recovery is really like. I do believe that the best part of my job is knowing the purpose behind the study. It is stated on our participants consent form. Simply it says, by your contribution of information it may help in changing things and help others to live a clean and sober life. I heard on a commercial for IBM recently that the collection of data is wisdom sharing, it is community. I strongly believe that this is the commitment this Center embodies. I hope the small part I play in this study contributes to the American community that wants to change how the disease of addiction is viewed and treated. We do recover!

By being a part of the team and a person in recovery it allowed me to see how fortunate I am. I witnessed first hand the struggles of individuals and most of all their families. I knew the hardships I caused but never realized the impact it had on the ones that love me. It helped me to understand the hurt and fear that the people in our lives have to endure. I say this not just as a person in recovery but as a person who today knows a little more because of my life experiences. Another thing that I thought was pretty cool was the fact that all you educated people at DePaul don't think that you're too good or above other people. I'm sure there was some doubt on your part as if this would all work out. But it did! I now have another family in my life, the DePaul Research Team.

The most obvious occurrence that has taken place in my life is that, I am now attending college full time at age 45. It is my belief that my association with the DePaul students and staff has motivated me to want to earn a degree. My involvement with the Oxford Study probably will be one of the most significant milestones in my life and for that I am truly grateful.

I've learned so many new terms which are used in the field of Psychology, and how to apply them to the work that I do as a recruiter on the Oxford House Research Project, that it has forced me to view recovery in supportive environments in a way one would not even be able to conceive, unless he or she had been afforded the opportunity to work in this particular atmosphere. It has also afforded me to work with a lot of caring, good people that have allowed me to be completely involved from start to finish in this thing; who listened when I had something to say, or an idea to present.

I have not experienced many major changes, except that my network of people that I know through Oxford House has grown.

DISCUSSION

The results indicated that the citizen collaborators from the Oxford House project generally felt positive about their experience with the research team as reflected by their ratings directionally improving. In fact, in six areas these improvements were statistically significant: communications, influence regarding research issues, influence regarding implementing the project, investment, knowledge about research methods, and feeling part of the team. It is also interesting that identification was about equal with DePaul and Oxford House at the start of the study, but by project end, the Oxford House recruiters were even more identified with Oxford House–this is an important finding as it indicates that the recruiters' association with the research team had not weakened or diminished their strong association with Oxford House. Findings clearly indicate that the Oxford House recruiters felt good about their collaboration with the research projects and the DePaul researchers.

However, unmistakably it was not merely their involvement but the recruiters' ability to communicate with and be heard by the university researchers and their trust in and impact on the research endeavor that contributed to the experience–for both the Oxford House members and researchers. Over the years of collaborative interaction, the research team has welcomed the expertise of the citizen recruiters and made many substantial revisions based upon their opinions. For example, in the NIDA study, the original study proposal stipulated that interviews to Oxford House members across the country would be conducted via telephone. However, based on feedback from members of Oxford House who worked with the research team, it was learned that residents were more willing to participate and would respond more openly to personal methods of data collection. Based on the recommendation of the Illinois recruiters and other Oxford House residents, it was decided to revise the proposed methodology and instead hire field-based Oxford House recruiters to visit houses and collect the data in person. Active involvement of the Oxford House members in the planning of the research methodology probably led to more favorable ratings related to being invested in the research effort and becoming more knowledgeable about research over time.

The Oxford House members of our team also constantly helped the researchers think about ways of sensitizing the interviews for this population. As an example, one question of the Addiction Severity Index inquires as to "What is the route of administration?" One of our Oxford House recruiters said that our participants would better understand this question if we just asked "How did you use it?" We simplified this question and when collecting these data, it was apparent that small changes such as this helped us obtain data that was not compromised by jargon used by researchers. Actively involving the Oxford House members in the implementation of the study probably led them to feel that they had a growing influence on the research process over time. The recruiters were aware of the research leaders' willingness to include members' input into the questions that were being analyzed, and this openness also contributed to the positive overall ratings and their feeling that the Oxford House perspective was being included within the overall study. The researchers also gained by the involvement of the Oxford House members. By involving participants in the design of the research, the researchers gained a greater appreciation of the culture and unique needs of the community. In addition, the researchers close association with the Oxford House organization facilitated their efforts to obtain funding at NIH.

There are several limitations in the present study. First, despite the fact that significant results suggested that the effects were robust, the sample size is extremely small. Second, there might have been demand characteristics that influenced the ratings, even though the respondents were told that the surveys would be culled anonymously and that their honest responses were requested and no negative reactions would occur regardless of their ratings. Third, it would have been better to have distributed the forms at the beginning of the employment with DePaul, rather than ask for a retrospective rating. Future research should employ such a design. It is also important to better document whether such attitudinal changes actually led to efforts by the community members to become more active in either research efforts or efforts to change the environment or political system. If community members become more knowledgeable and empowered as a function of participating on these types of research efforts, it is important to assess whether the community members bring their new insights, skills and resources to the resolution of issues in their own communities (Ferrari & Jason, 1996).

Citizen participation can mean simply agreeing to take part in a study, providing staff support from a community organization, actively collaborating in study implementation, or simply having veto power at any time (Jason et al., 2004). Participation can also occur at different phases of the research investigation, from generating the original idea, through planning the design, carrying out the data collection, and/or implementing the results. Regardless of how participation is defined, it is important to better assess the impact of this participation on the citizens and community members who are involved in the research effort.

REFERENCES

Chataway, C. J. (2001). Negotiating the observer-observed relationship: Participatory action research. In D. Tolman and M. Brydon-Miller (Eds.), *From subjects to subjectivities: A handbook of interpretive and participatory methods* (239-255). New York: New York University Press.

Ferrari, J. R., & Jason, L. A. (1996). Integrating research and community service: Incorporating research skills into service learning experiences. *College Student Journal, 30*, 444-451.

Jason, L. A., Davis, M. I., Suarez-Balcazar, Y., Keys, C. B., Taylor, R. R., Holtz Isenberg, D., & Durlak, J. (2004). Conclusion. In L. A. Jason, C. B. Keys, Y. Suarez-Balcazar, R. R. Taylor, M. Davis, J. Durlak, & D. Isenberg (Eds.). *Participatory community research: Theories and methods in action.* American Psychological Association: Washington, D.C.

Jason, L. A., Ferrari, J. R., Smith, B., Marsh, P. Dvorchak, P. A., Groessl, E. K., Pechota, M. E., Curtin, M. E., Bishop, P. D., Grams, G., Kot, E., & Bowden, B. S. (1997). An exploratory study of male recovering substance abusers living in a self-help, self-governed setting. *Journal of Mental Health Administration, 24*, 332-339.

Jason, L. A., & Glenwick, D. S. (Eds.) (2002). *Innovative strategies for promoting health and mental health across the lifespan.* New York, NY: Springer Publishing.

Keiffer, J. G. (1984). Citizen empowerment: A developmental perspective. *Prevention in Human Services, 3*, 9-36.

Kelly, J. G. (1990). Changing contexts and the field of community psychology. *American Journal of Community Psychology, 18*, 769-792.

Montgomery, H. A., Miller, W. R., & Tonigan, J. S. (1993). Differences among AA groups: Implications for research. *Journal of Studies on Alcohol, 54*, 502-504.

Wandersman, A., Chavis, D., & Stucky, P. (1983). Involving citizens in research. In R. Kidd and M. Saks (Eds.), *Advances in applied social psychology* (pp.189-212). Hillsdale, NJ: Erlbaum.

PART 2:
RESIDENCE FOR RECOVERY

Chapter 3:
Creating a Home to Promote Recovery:
The Physical Environments
of Oxford House

Joseph R. Ferrari
Leonard A. Jason
Kelly C. Sasser

DePaul University

Margaret I. Davis

Dickinson College

Bradley D. Olson

DePaul University

The authors express much gratitude to the Oxford House members who allowed them to visit their homes and conduct their observations, and to Robin Miller, Bill Kmeck, Kathy Erikson, Bertell Williams, Joe Chavez, and Gregory Corscadden for collecting data and result feedback.

Funding for this manuscript was made possible in part by NIH grant awards from the National Institute for Alcohol and Alcohol Abuse (NIAAA # AA12218) and National Institute on Drug Abuse (NIDA # DA13231). Portions of these results were reported in a DePaul Senior Honor's Thesis by Kelly C. Sasser under the supervision of Joseph R. Ferrari and Leonard A. Jason, and presented at the 2001 *Eastern Psychological Association* meeting (Boston, MA).

[Haworth co-indexing entry note]: "Chapter 3: Creating a Home to Promote Recovery: The Physical Environments of Oxford House." Ferrari, Joseph R. et al. Co-published simultaneously in *Journal of Prevention & Intervention in the Community* (The Haworth Press, Inc.) Vol. 31, No.1/2, 2006, pp. 27-39; and: *Creating Communities for Addiction Recovery: The Oxford House Model* (ed: Jason et al.) The Haworth Press, Inc., 2006, pp. 27-39. Single or multiple copies of this article are available for a fee from The Haworth Document Delivery Service [1-800-HAWORTH, 9:00 a.m. - 5:00 p.m. (EST). E-mail address: docdelivery@haworthpress.com].

Available online at http://www.haworthpress.com/web/JPIC
doi:10.1300/J005v31n01_03

SUMMARY. The interior and exterior physical characteristics of substance abuse recovery program dwellings (11 women, 44 men) from three geographic sections of the United States were assessed as creating a "house-as-home" for residents. Although each house was independently governed and operated by residents, results indicated vast similarities among the interior characteristics, amenities, and structural aspects. These rented dwellings also had similar well-maintained exterior characteristics, despite their geographic locations. Follow-up interviews of former residents indicated that these house characteristics and amenities helped create a sense of home not found in traditional institutional facilities. Results suggested that residents of self-governed independently operated recovery houses may create and maintain safe and sober settings that elicit a sense of home among residents. *[Article copies available for a fee from The Haworth Document Delivery Service: 1-800-HAWORTH. E-mail address: <docdelivery@haworthpress.com> Website: <http://www.HaworthPress.com>* © 2006 by The Haworth Press, Inc. All rights reserved.]*

KEYWORDS. Oxford House, house-as-home, physical interior and exterior

"A place called home"–what does that expression mean? Smith (1994a; 1994b) found that for married and "living-together" couples a sense of "home" included performing chores with each other, social interactions over personal and professional issues, and sharing in recreational activities. Moreover, a sense of home included being able, within a physical structure, to self-express one's personal identity. Smith reported that physical artifacts expressing personal identity created a sense of "home" as a warm, at-peace, security dwelling. A strong sense of *psychological home* may prompt a person to modify a setting through exterior and interior design that better reflects the identity of a person (Sigmon, Whitcomb, & Snyder, 2002), a reflection of the person's "house-as-a-symbol of self" (Cooper, 1974).

Traditionally, psychologists examined a variable labeled a *sense of community*: identification with, or sense of belonging, to a group of individuals often tied to a specific geographic location (see Fisher, Sonn, & Bishop, 2002). A person's psychological home differs from a sense of community in that "home" is related to how an individual expresses self-identity in one or more physical environments. Psychological home is a person's need to express his/her self-identity, often in physical settings, but independent from any specific social group. For instance, a person may choose to place family pictures and personal artifacts reflective of their family around their office and in their car, to make themselves feel at home. Although different than a sense of community, a person's psychological home may be strengthened by the social support and positive interactions he/she experiences with others (Smith, 1994a; 1994b). A supportive social network may enhance a person's freedom of self-expression by establishing a safe haven (Sigmon et al., 2002).

In the present study, we focused on the safe and sober settings persons in recovery from drug and alcohol addiction created as "home." Traditional substance abuse treatment facilities include dwellings where many residents share bedrooms and common spaces with several other residents but often do not have opportunities for close interpersonal contact that fosters a sense of community among persons. Residents in traditional treatment settings are not expected to personally contribute funds to operate the site because government and/or insurance programs cover costs. Furthermore, treatment costs are considerable given the salaries of trained professionals who operate the site and plant managers who maintain the physical grounds. Treatment programs at traditional sites may contribute to the lack of connectedness among residents by staff-mandated rules and regulations, where residents had little or no input in self-governance.

Consequently, there is a tremendous need to develop, evaluate and expand low cost, non-medical, community-based care options for substance abuse patients (Jason, Olson, Ferrari, & Davis, 2004; Ferrari, Jason, Olson, Davis, & Alvarez, 2002). The present study presented an overview and assessment of *Oxford House*, a network of homes that offers residents a supportive, democratic, mutual-help setting, established, governed, and maintained by recovering substance abusers living together to develop long-term abstinence skills. We believe that these abstinent supportive communal settings create for residents the "family" like atmosphere reflective of a "home." Consistent with Smith (1994a; 1994b), sharing chores, social interactions, and recreational activities among members of an Oxford House may contribute to the sense of home that they create. Furthermore, living in a "home" with similar peers who are like "family" may promote for persons in recovery from addiction the belief that they can maintain sobriety even under adverse conditions.

Research on the Oxford House recovery model found that self-governance within a communal-living "family" environment is appropriate for diverse populations (Alvarez, Jason, Olson, Ferrari, & Davis, 2003;

Ferrari, Curtin, Dvorchak, & Jason, 1997; Ferrari, Jason et al., 1999; Majer, Jason, Ferrari, Venable, & Olson, 2001). This fact is important, for instance, given that women and women with children in recovery have needs frequently unmet by conventional treatment programs (Dvorchak, Grams, Tate, & Jason, 1995; Ferrari et al., 1997). The benefits of the "home" environment of an Oxford House also has been an attractive alternative for African-Americans (Ferrari et al., 1997), as well as women with personal histories of trauma and physical abuse (Olson, Curtis, Jason, Ferrari et al., 2003). Men and women residents maintain employment, thereby reducing the need for government subsidies and interventions (Jason, Ferrari, Smith et al., 1997). At present, there are over 1,000 U.S., 35 Canadian, and 6 Australian Oxford Houses (Paul Molloy, personal communication, May 2004) providing a place for men, women, women with children, and even men with children (see d'Arlach, Curtis, Ferrari, Olson, & Jason, in press; Ferrari et al., 1999).

Ferrari et al. (2002) noted that in Oxford House residents build a sense of community from sharing experiences and learning skills from other residents. We believe that this mutual supportive environment contributed to the autonomy that facilitates recovery within Oxford House. The sense of community residents develop in an Oxford House may complement and facilitate the development of a sense of "home" within the House. Residents of Oxford House may feel empowered to engage in self-expression of their personal identity, by decorating the interior and/or exterior of the dwelling. Understanding a person's sense of home includes examining the characteristics of a suitable physical structure (interior and exterior) that may contribute to the emotional reactions and expression of personal identity (Smith, 1994a). Despite previous evaluations of Oxford House, the present study is the first detailed assembly on the interior and exterior physical environment of these independent "homes."

METHOD

Sites and Residents

We evaluated 11 women and 44 men Oxford Houses operating as of 2002 along the east coast (Virginia: 2 women, 16 men), mid-west (Illinois: 5 women, 16 men), and west coast (Hawaii: 4 women, 12 men) of the United States. Each House was a single-family, residential dwelling rented by 6 to 8 residents (M number = 7.6). These three geographic regions provided an overview of residence characteristics from three clearly different and independent sections of "Americana." Most residents were European-American (68.8%), although over 90% of these 55 Houses had at least one resident of color (typically, African-American). On average, the blocks for each House had 19.9 other homes. Consistent with the Oxford House model, these Houses typically were usually located in suburban neighborhoods (77.3%) and in "working-class" communities (59.3%).

Procedure

Our research team initially discussed the observation items used for this assessment with Oxford House officials. Two observers then independently visited all 21 Illinois Oxford Houses, recording the interior and exterior of each setting. Two other observers visited 18 Virginia and 16 Hawaii Oxford Houses. Observations from leaders at these Houses were used to calculate inter-observer reliability from independent assessments. Inter-observer reliability ranged from 94-99% agreement between observers across sites. It took approximately one month to collect the Illinois data and three months for the information from Hawaii and Virginia.

At each dwelling, an observer completed a survey on the interior and exterior House characteristics plus immediate surroundings of the House. Each observer walked throughout the house and checked off all the items found from a list of physical objects. The House interior items observed included: beds, toilets, showers, tubs, desks, dressers, lamps, mirrors, large public areas, air conditioners, locked bathrooms, pictures on the walls, plants/decorations on windowsills, handrails, TV family rooms, comfortable furniture, microwaves, working kitchen appliances, and no smoking areas. Subsequently, we asked 3 women and 4 men who lived in an Oxford House how the results fit with their experiences of a "house-as-home." We included a paraphrase of these comments from Oxford House "alumni" whom had recent access with the Houses on how the interior and exterior amenities observed make the setting a home. We did not choose current residents because we wanted unobtrusive assessments of these Houses.

RESULTS AND DISCUSSION

Our presentation on the "typical Oxford House" across the United States included the physical interior and exterior of our sample dwellings to visualize what an average House may look like and understand how residents created a physical structure for self-expression of their identity (Smith, 1994a). *Chi square* and one-way *ANOVAs* (controlling for Type 1 errors) compared setting characteristics across sites.

House Interior Profile

Table 1 presents the average number or percentage of items observed inside Virginia, Illinois, and Hawaii Houses. There were significant differences in the number of bedrooms found across the three geographic sites, $F(2, 54) = 8.32$, $p < .01$, with more bedrooms in Virginia than Illinois or Hawaii Houses. Virginia also had significantly more bedroom desks than Illinois or Hawaii Houses, $F(2, 54) = 17.18$, $p < .001$, and more bedroom lamps than Hawaii Houses, $F(2, 54) = 12.93$, $p < .003$, but similar number of bedroom mirrors was found across all three sites of Houses. Virginia Houses, however, had significantly fewer large communal areas for residents that Illinois or Hawaii Houses $F(2, 54) = 5.66$, $p < .006$. There also were significant differences across states in the number of toilets, $F(2, 54) = 6.15$, $p < .004$, and showers $F(2, 54) = 30.19$, $p < .001$, although the number of tubs was similar across the three sites. These results may reflect dwelling differences attributive to the size of the House rather than the location of the Houses. That is, because Virginia Houses have more bedrooms than the other states they may have less square footage to devote to communal living spaces such as living rooms and family rooms.

We also observed whether the Houses in our sample had other conveniences within the interior of the residence. There were significant differences in the presence of only a few interior items observed, namely: planters on windowsills, $\chi^2(2; n = 53) = 12.25$, $p < .002$, working appliances in kitchens, $\chi^2(2; n = 53) = 12.06$, $p < .002$, and established non-smoking areas within the House, $\chi^2(2; n = 53) = 12.25$, $p < .001$. Hawaii Houses had lowest percentages of dwellings with windowsill planters and functioning kitchen appliances, and Illinois Houses had the highest percentage of interior non-smoking areas across the three geographic areas. Regardless of geographic location, most Oxford Houses had personal dressers in each bedroom (96.2%), room air-conditioners (70.9%), a utility room or designated space for laundry (96.2%), rooms decorated with pictures on the wall (100%), safety handrails on stairways (77.4%), communal lounges with televisions (98.1%), public

TABLE 1. Mean Number or Percentage of Presence of Characteristics Observed Inside an Oxford House

	OXFORD HOUSE LOCATIONS		
	VIRGINIA	ILLINOIS	HAWAII
HOUSE INTERIOR:	(n = 18)	(n = 21)	(n =16)
Average number of…			
Bedrooms	7.06^{a,b}	5.62^a	5.38^b
Bedroom desks	3.78^{b,c}	1.29^{a,b}	2.37^{a,c}
Bedroom lamps	6.44^a	5.24	3.63^a
Bedroom mirrors	2.89	1.81	2.69
Large public areas	3.94^{a,b}	4.71^a	5.13^b
Bathrooms (toilets)	3.11^b	2.14^{a,b}	2.82^a
Tubs with showers	1.50	1.43	1.69
Shower only	2.06^b	0.24^{a,b}	1.63^a
Proportion of Houses (%) with …			
Personal dressers	94.4	94.7	100
Room air-conditioners	67.8	69.2	74.8
Laundry room/space	100	100	87.5
Locked bathroom doors	83.3	52.6	93.8
Pictures on walls	100	100	100
Plants on windowsills	72.2^{b,c}	47.4^{a,b}	12.5^{a,c}
Handrails on stairs	83.3	89.5	56.3
Communal lounge with TV	94.4	100	100
Communal telephone	100	100	100
Comfortable communal furniture	100	100	100
Working kitchen appliances	94.4^{b,c}	89.5^{a,b}	50.0^{a,c}
Microwave in kitchen	100	100	100
Non-smoking area	16.7^{b,c}	100^{a,c}	50.0^{a,b}

Note. [a,b,c] Values with similar superscripts are significantly different.

accessible telephones (100%), comfortable communal furniture (100%), and a functioning microwave (100%).

House Interiors: Former Resident Perspective. Persons who once lived in an Oxford House told us that offering residents their own bedroom contributed to a sense of home. One person stated that, as an adult, when he shared his bedroom with another person in a traditional treatment facility, he did not feel that the room was his home— it had an institutional feeling. Unlike institutional facilities, these persons claimed that large communal spaces in an Oxford House (such as a dining room or a family room) fostered interactions among residents.

Another person noted that having her own dresser for personal items gave her a feeling that Oxford House was home, and another person stated that having a laundry facility on site permitted her to feel comfortable in the Oxford House making the dwelling feel like "home." Decorating the House with personal possessions was another opportunity that the Oxford House experience provided residents. In one man's House a new (inexpensive) blind was purchased each year to update and refresh the "home" atmosphere. One person commented that when his grandmother died he furnished his House with her furniture including a painting that he always admired that was hung in the living room. Seeing that painting on a daily basis in his "home" was an opportunity he never experienced living in previous institutional facilities. Having flowers on windowsills and plants around the house added to a sense of home, unlike their experiences in institutional settings where they had been before where there were no flowers or plants inside the facility.

Taken together, the interior characteristics of Oxford House dwellings noted in three different geographic locations across the United States complement the personal reflections on the interior characteristics of Oxford Houses. When given the opportunity to create their own living environment, Oxford House residents created a "home" with comfort items and conveniences (Smith, 1994b). We believe this fact demonstrates that persons in recovery, even when separated from biological family members, may create a home atmosphere when given the opportunity to self-govern their life living with peers.

House Exterior Profiles

Table 2 presents the mean number or percentage of house exterior and neighbor physical characteristics across states on Oxford Houses. There were significant differences across the three geographic locations on the number of house exterior items observed. Specifically, Illinois Houses in comparison to the other two sites had significantly more flaking of dwelling paint or siding, $F(2, 53) = 16.19$, $p < .001$, neighboring homes were found with broken windows or screen door, $F(2, 53) = 5.26$, $p < .009$, yards with litter, $F(2, 53) = 24.18$, $p < .001$, and potholes on the street, $F(2, 53) = 9.81$, $p < .001$. Illinois Houses had significantly more vacancy signs for rental or sale properties, $F(2, 53) = 5.64$, $p < .006$, than at the other sites. However, across sites there were not many dwellings with graffiti on the residence, overgrown bushes or grass in the front yards, abandoned houses, vacant lots, or cracking sidewalks (see Table 2).

We noted few significant differences in other exterior characteristics from this Oxford House sample (see Table 2). These differences included: presence of a front doorbell, $\chi^2(2, n = 53) = 11.03$, $p < .004$, a formal outdoor patio or courtyard, $\chi^2(2, n = 53) = 6.93$, $p < .003$, and a flower or vegetable garden, $\chi^2(2, n = 53) = 17.78$, $p < .001$. There were a lower percentage of a front door bell yet higher percentage of a patio or courtyard with Hawaii Houses, and a significant difference across the three sites on the presence of a flower/vegetable garden with the percentage of Illinois Houses having the fewest. In contrast, most Oxford Houses had a shelter covering over the front entrance doorway to protect persons from inclement weather (69.8%), only a front door as access to the House (84.6%), outdoor yard furniture (50.9%) and an outdoor barbeque for cooking (81.1%), a grassy lawn (86.8%), outdoor lights to use at night for security (92.5%), and a communal mailbox for postal delivery (82.4%).

House Exterior: Former Resident's Perspective. The "alumni" residents stated that having a patio or courtyard, outdoor furniture, a barbeque, and a lawn made their Oxford House feel "homey." These exterior House amenities provided opportunities for residents to meet, talk, perhaps share a meal, and get to know each other in a comfortable, informal setting where they lived. One person indicated that the annual planting and harvesting of vegetables was a communal activity that created pride in having a "home." Unlike traditional institutions where a paid superintendent controls maintenance, there was a sense of pride in maintaining their Oxford House to "look good," even though they were not the owners of the dwelling.

We believe the differences observed on exterior characteristics may be attributed to where the Houses were located. The Illinois Oxford Houses were located in more urban settings than either the Virginia or Hawaii Houses, which may explain the higher number of potholes in the

TABLE 2. Mean Number or Percentage of Presence of Characteristics Observed Outside an Oxford House

	OXFORD HOUSE LOCATIONS		
	VIRGINIA	ILLINOIS	HAWAII
HOUSE EXTERIOR:	(n = 18)	(n = 21)	(n = 16)
Average number of…			
flaking paint/bare wood/siding:	.72[b]	3.11[a,b]	.19[a]
broken windows/screen doors	.39[b]	.78[a,b]	0[a]
graffiti on house, wall	.13	.23	.13
overgrown bushes or grass	.94	1.22	.69
abandoned cars/appliances in yard	.78	.22	.81
yards with litter	.44[b]	2.11[a,b]	.19[a]
abandoned houses on block	.11	.28	0
vacancy signs (rent, sale)	.56[b,c]	.83[a,b]	.19[a,c]
vacant lots	0	0	.10
sidewalks with cracks	1.67	3.22	1.38
potholes	1.89[b]	3.22[a,b]	.50[a]
Proportion of Houses (%) with …			
Shelter over front door	77.8	52.6	81.6
Front door access only	76.7	89.5	87.5
Front doorbell	28.1[b]	53.1[a,b]	18.8[a]
Patio/courtyard	83.3[b]	57.9[a,b]	93.8[a]
Outdoor furniture	66.7	36.8	50.0
Outdoor barbeque	72.2	89.5	81.3
Flower/vegetable garden	83.3[a,b]	15.8[b,c]	62.5[a,c]
Lawn	88.9	84.2	87.5
Outdoor night-lights	100	89.5	87.5
Mailbox	72.8	100	74.9

Note. Values with similar superscripts are significantly different.

streets. Possibly, the dwellings rented as Oxford Houses in Illinois were available only on blocks where there was more transition in ownership, explaining the higher number of vacancy signs than the other two locations. Because all Houses were rented, the Illinois Houses may have been established in more affordable neighborhoods that seemed a bit more "worn" and unattractive than Virginia or Hawaii, suggesting the reason for the observed flaking of house paint, broken windows, and yard litter. Results found that the exterior characteristics of Oxford Houses were very similar in amenities (e.g., mailboxes, barbeques, and lawns). When taken together with the vast similarities observed on the interior characteristics, our results on exterior characteristics of Oxford House suggest that despite a few neighborhood differences, residents of Oxford House made their house a home. Finding affordable, attractive housing for persons recovering from addictions may be difficult, yet the residents of Oxford House created a safe and sober "house-as-home."

In summary, this study indicated that Oxford House residents who live in a community of abstinent others make their "house" a "home." Across three diverse regions of the United States, Oxford House residents lived in rather similar dwellings, a setting that looked and felt like a home. Interviews of persons who once lived in an Oxford House added depth to the statistical results: the voices of those persons were consistent with what was observed across sites. The present study suggested that shared activities that occur within an Oxford House, such as chores, social activities, BBQs, watching TV, and gatherings on outdoor decks and patios, may help residents create a sense of community with other members. Engaging in pleasant, constructive activities builds a connectedness with other members.

Moreover, the sense of community that Oxford House residents experience may complement the development of a sense of home that each resident may experience. Consistent with other studies (e.g., Sigmon et al., 2002; Smith 1994a, 1994b), a person's psychological home includes a secure, warm, positive feeling where self-expression is permitted and a feeling of belongingness with others both exist. The physical amenities inside and outside a house, along with the freedom to personally express themselves by decorating and structuring the house, gives residents personal pride and self-affirmation of their individuality, adding to a *sense of home*.

REFERENCES

Alvarez, J., Jason, L. A., Olson, B. D., Ferrari, J. R., & Davis, M. I. (2003). *A review of substance use and abuse among Latinos and Latinas.* Manuscript under review.

Cooper, C. (1974). The house as symbol of the self. In J. Lang (Ed.). *Designing for human behavior.* Stroudsburg, PA: Dowden, Hutchinson, & Ross.

d'Arlach, L., Curtis, C. E., Ferrari, J. R., Olson, B.D., & Jason, L.A. (in press). Substance-abuse women and children: Cost-effective treatment options. *Journal of Social Work Practice in the Addictions.*

Dvorchak, P., Grams, G., Tate, L., & Jason, L. A. (1995). Pregnant and post-partum women in recovery: Barriers to treatment and the role of Oxford House in the continuation of care. *Alcohol Treatment Quarterly, 13,* 97-107.

Ferrari, J. R., Curtin, M., Dvorchak, P., & Jason, L. A. (1997). Recovering from alcoholism in communal-living settings: Exploring characteristics of African-American men and women. *Journal of Substance Abuse, 9,* 77-87.

Ferrari, J. R., Jason, L. A., Nelson, R., Curtin-Davis, M., Marsh, P., & Smith, B. (1999). An exploratory analysis of women and men within self-help, communal-living recovery settings: A new beginning in a new house. *American Journal of Drug and Alcohol Abuse, 25,* 305-317.

Fisher, A. T., Sonn, C.C., & Bishop, B. J. (2002). *Psychological sense of community: Research, applications, and implications.* New York: Kluwer Academic/Plenum Publications.

Jason, L. A., Davis, M. I., Ferrari, J. R., & Bishop, P. (2001). Oxford House: A review of research and implications for substance abuse recovery and community research. *Journal of Drug Education, 31,* 1-27.

Jason, L. A., Ferrari, J. R., Dvorchak, P. A., Groessl, E. J., & Molloy, J. P. (1997). The characteristics of alcoholics in self-help residential treatment settings: A multi-site study of Oxford House. *Alcoholism Treatment Quarterly, 15,* 53-63.

Jason, L. A., Ferrari, J. R., Smith, B., Marsh, P., Dvorchak, P. A., Groessl, E., Pechota, M. E., Curtin, M., Bishop, P. D., Grams, G., Kot, E., & Bowden, B.S. (1997). An exploratory study of male recovering substance abusers living in a self-help, self-governed setting. *Journal of Mental Health Administration, 24,* 332-339.

Jason, L. A., Olson, B. D., Ferrari, J. R., & Davis, M. I. (2004). Substance abuse: The need for second order change. *International Journal of Self-Help and Self-Care, 2,* 91-109.

Jason, L. A., Pechota, Bowden, B. S., Lahmar, K., Pokorny, S., Bishop, P., Quintana, E., Sangerman, C., Salina, D., Taylor, S., Lesondak, L., & Grams, G. (1994). Oxford House: Community living is community healing. *Addictions: Concepts and strategies for treatment.* (pp. 333-338). Gaithersburg, MD: Aspen.

Nealon-Woods, M.A., Ferrari, J. R., & Ferrari, L. A. (1995). Twelve-step program use among Oxford House residents: Spirituality vs. social support in sobriety. *Journal of Substance Abuse, 7,* 311-318.

Olson, B. D., Curtis, C. E., Jason, L. A., Ferrari, J. R., Horin, E. V., Davis, M. I., Flynn, A.M., & Alvarez, J. (2003). Physical and sexual trauma among women in substance abuse recovery: Suggestions for a new model of shelter aftercare. *Journal of Prevention & Intervention in the Community, 26,* 67-80.

Oxford House, Inc. (1988). *Oxford House Manual.* Silver Spring, MD.

Sigmon, S. T., Whitcomb, S. R., & Snyder, C. R. (2002). Psychological home. In A.T. Fisher, C.S. Sonn, & B.J. Bishop (Eds.), pp. 25-41, *Psychological sense of community: Research, applications, and implications.* New York: Kluwer/Plenum Publications.

Smith, S.G. (1994a). The essential qualities of home. *Journal of Environmental Psychology, 14,* 31-46.

Smith, S.G. (1994b). The psychological construction of home life. *Journal of Environmental Psychology, 14,* 125-136.

Chapter 4:
"This Is My Neighborhood":
Comparing United States and Australian
Oxford House Neighborhoods

Joseph R. Ferrari
Leonard A. Jason

DePaul University

Ron Blake

Oxford House, Australia

Margaret I. Davis

Dickinson College

Bradley D. Olson

DePaul University

Address correspondence to: Joseph R. Ferrari, Department of Psychology, DePaul University, 2219 North Kenmore Avenue, Chicago, IL 60614 (E-mail: jferrari@ depaul. edu).

The authors express much gratitude to the Oxford House members who allowed visits to their homes and to Kelly Sassar, Kathy Erikson, Bertell Williams (Illinois), Joe Chavez (Hawaii), and Gregory Corscadden (Virginia) for data collection.

Funding for this manuscript was made possible in part by NIH grant awards from National Institute for Alcohol and Alcohol Abuse (NIAAA # AA12218) and National Institute on Drug Abuse (NIDA # DA13231).

[Haworth co-indexing entry note]: "Chapter 4: "This Is My Neighborhood": Comparing United States and Australian Oxford House Neighborhoods." Ferrari, Joseph R. et al. Co-published simultaneously in *Journal of Prevention & Intervention in the Community* (The Haworth Press, Inc.) Vol. 31, No.1/2, 2006, pp. 41-49; and: *Creating Communities for Addiction Recovery: The Oxford House Model* (ed: Jason et al.) The Haworth Press, Inc., 2006, pp. 41-49. Single or multiple copies of this article are available for a fee from The Haworth Document Delivery Service [1-800-HAWORTH, 9:00 a.m. - 5:00 p.m. (EST). E-mail address: docdelivery@ haworthpress.com].

41

SUMMARY. The number of Oxford Houses, communal-living, mutual help settings for persons in recovery of alcohol and substance abuse, has spread across the United States and recently in and around Melbourne, Australia. In this study 55 US and 6 AU Houses were compared descriptively for their neighborhood characteristics. Across settings, there were greater similarities than significant differences in the locations. Results imply that Australian Oxford Houses are "safe and sober" settings for persons in recovery consistent with the original United States model in physical dwelling settings. *[Article copies available for a fee from The Haworth Document Delivery Service: 1-800-HAWORTH. E-mail address: <docdelivery@haworthpress.com> Website: <http://www.HaworthPress.com>* © 2006 by The Haworth Press, Inc. All rights reserved.]

KEYWORDS. Oxford House, Australia, neighborhood characteristics, physical settings

In the novel *Of Mice and Men,* by John Steinbeck, the author describes the bunkhouse where the migrant workers sleep. Each man is given a used mattress to sleep on, but attached to the wall is their personal box for belongings and items, held by an old wood crate. To these workers, their home lay inside that box–that box/shelf represented their home. In the Beach Boys' classic song from the 1960s, *In My Room,* a teenager's bedroom is described where he can shut out the world and focus on his own life away from adults and the troubles in growing up. When talking about the mobility of their sense of home, a couple might say "wherever we're together that's my home." The couple feels at home in any location because they experience a feeling of security and the ability to express their self as an individual. A person's home reflects his/her sense of identity regardless of the physical dwelling–a "house-as-a-symbol of self" (Cooper, 1974; Sigmon, Whitcomb, & Snyder, 2002).

In the present study we assessed *Oxford House,* a network of homes that offer residents a supportive, democratic, mutual-help setting, established and maintained by recovering substance abusers living together to develop long-term abstinence skills. *Oxford House* was founded in 1975 by Paul Molloy and a group of peers who were recovering from alcoholism. These pioneers voted to repeal several cornerstone rules common to treatment facilities: 6-month restriction on length of stay, curfews, and numerous staff-imposed rules. Instead, they established only a few fundamental rules that remain today: (1) residents of each

House must remain abstinent from alcohol and other drugs; (2) each House must maintain financial independence by residents paying their equal share of the rent and operating costs; (3) House residents accept responsibility for doing specific house chores; (4) each House resident must not be disruptive or cause harm to other residents; and, (5) each House must be democratically operated by the residents of that dwelling (i.e., > 80% approval rate). Deviations from financial responsibilities to the House, disruptive, anti-social behaviors, or resuming drugs or alcohol use result in eviction (Jason, Ferrari, Dvorchak, Groessl, & Molloy, 1997; Oxford House Manual, 1998). Ferrari, Jason, Davis, Olson, and Alvarez (2004) reported that across the United States these Houses used similar self-governed policies and liberties among residents that were more democratic than traditional therapeutic communities.

In 1988, the Anti-Drug Abuse Act passed by the U.S. Congress allocated federal funds to any state for the start-up of Oxford Houses. A group of recovering substance abusers, through the support of an established House, may request only $4,000 from their state in an interest-free loan to begin a new Oxford House. Repayment of loans is returned to the fund for start-up costs of additional Houses in that state. These rented Houses are multi-bedroom dwellings for same-sex occupants (range = 6-8 persons). At present, 70% are male Houses and 30% are female Houses; 55% of occupants are Caucasian, 35% are African-American, 5% are Hispanic, and 5% are other (e.g., Asian-Americans). The number of Oxford Houses replicating this community-based model for substance abuse recovery has increased to nearly 1000 within the United States (Paul Molloy, personal communication, May 2004).

ASSESSING THE NEIGHBORHOOD ENVIRONMENT OF OXFORD HOUSES: AN EXPLORATORY STUDY

Oxford House residents seek a safe, clean, and affordable housing environment to call *home*. Ferrari, Jason, Sasser, Davis, and Olson (2006) found from three geographic sections of the United States that Oxford Houses were very similar both in interior living space and exterior upkeep. Former residents felt that their House had a strong "homey" feeling because of the physical artifacts, decorating, and amenities the residents developed in the dwelling. Jason, Roberts, and Olson (2004) found that neighbors living in immediate proximity of a U.S. Oxford House considered the residents more positively than persons living blocks away; moreover, property values on the block where Houses were located did not decrease once the setting was established.

Despite our pilot and on-going evaluations of Oxford House across the United States, the present study is the first detailed assembly on the neighborhood setting characteristics of Oxford House. We believe that to understand a persons' sense of home, one also needs to appreciate the neighborhood setting for that dwelling. Because each Oxford House attempts to operate within a part of its local community so residents learn about and gain access to local resources, it is important to gain an understanding of the neighborhood characteristics. Furthermore, because the Oxford House concept now appears in international settings, we decided to include similar information on the small sample of existing Australian Oxford Houses. This information provides some insight into how global the Oxford House models to create safe and sober settings for persons in recovery has been implemented. We did not conduct any statistical analyses for gender or country differences between Houses, because our goal was to provide descriptive information on these communal-living settings and the sample sizes were so skewed biasing results.

A Sample of U.S. and Australian Oxford Houses

We evaluated 44 men and 11 women U.S. Oxford Houses operating along the east coast (Virginia: 2 women, 16 men), mid-west (Illinois: 5 women, 16 men), and west coast (Hawaii: 4 women, 12 men), as well as 5 men and 1 women Australian House from the state of Victoria (i.e., Melbourne area). We choose these three U.S. geographic regions in order to ascertain immediate neighborhood characteristics from three clearly different and independent sections of "Americana" and because there are only 6 Houses in Australia at the time of data collection in 2002-03. Each House was a single-family, residential dwelling with seven to eight residents (M number = 7.6) at the time of this project. Most residents were European-American (68.8%), although over 90% of the 55 U.S. Houses had at least one person of color (typically, African-American) resident. On average, the blocks for each House had about 20-23 other houses. Consistent with the Oxford House model, these Houses were usually located in suburban neighborhoods (73%) and in "working, middle class" communities (55%).

Data Collection Process. Initially, we discussed the neighborhood and setting characteristics items for this assessment with U.S. Oxford House officials and then pilot tested items while networking with residents from Illinois Oxford Houses to help shape the final battery of items. Subsequently, we trained alumni of Oxford House in the U.S. and the third author in Australia to observe in pairs the interior, exterior, and neighborhood characteristics of a House. Details on the observation process and items may be found in Ferrari et al. (2004, 2006). Inter-observer reliability ranged from 94-97% agreement between observers. It took approximately one to three months to collect the data across sites.

Survey Items. For each setting, an observer "walked around the block" and in close proximity to the House's neighborhood. We asked observers to judge whether the general surroundings seemed to be: economically depressed, accessible by public transportation, streets clean of litter, streets well lit at night, streets well kept, streets lined with trees and greenery, places for intoxicated/drug persons, drug dealers, or homeless persons, and easily accessible to pawn shops or pubs/bars selling alcohol. Finally, observers noted whether there were neighborhood amenities available for local residents. These amenities included: grocery stores, drug stores, movie theatre, church/synagogue, public library, bank, hospital, medical clinic, physician office, dentist office, post office, and park(s).

Results from Neighborhood Observations: U.S. and Australia. In creating a "house as home" for persons in recovery one must include an understanding of the neighborhood where that dwelling is located. Our focus was on the actual residence persons living in an Oxford House created as their home. Because of the large number of items recorded and the possibility of statistical errors in multiple analyses with such small sample sizes (e.g., only 6 Australian Houses), no statistical analyses on the neighborhood characteristics were performed. In fact, we found no meaningful differences across the three geographic U.S. settings on the few general surrounding neighborhood characteristics and amenities we did analyze using *chi square* analyses. Tables 1 and 2 presents the percentage of neighborhood characteristics the observers noted within a half-mile radius across the 6 Australian and 55 U.S. Oxford Houses assessed in this study. This information provides a profile and context for how an Oxford House "fits-in" to different neighborhoods in both countries.

General Surroundings. As noted from Table 1, both Australian and U.S. 55 Houses were generally located in rather economically enriched settings, where very few intoxicated persons or drug dealers were seen on the streets and no homeless persons found. The observers noted that public transportation generally was available, and the streets and neighborhoods were clean, well lit at night, and usually had trees and greenery.

TABLE 1. Percentage of Neighborhood Characteristics Within a Half-Mile of Oxford House

	OXFORD HOUSES	
	Australia	*United States*
	(n = 6)	*(n = 55)*
GENERAL SURROUNDINGS:		
economically depressed	0.0	11.7
intoxicated/drug person present	0.0	1.9
drug dealer present	0.0	3.8
homeless person–sleeping nearby	0.0	0.0
homeless person–present	0.0	0.0
neighborhood well kept	100	79.2
public transportation	100	83.7
streets clean/litter free	100	86.9
streets well lit	100	88.5
trees/greenery present	100	71.8
pawn shop nearby	0.0	5.8
empty lots present	0.0	25.4
bars/pubs nearby	33.3	30.0

Note. U.S. data include all Houses surveyed in Virginia, Illinois, and Hawaii.

While Australian and U.S. Houses usually did not have pawn shops nearby, there seemed to be a few more empty lots around U.S. Houses. Also, bars/pubs were nearby about a third of both Australian and U.S. Houses.

Neighborhood Amenities. Table 2 indicates that observers noted that within an easy commute around each House, many civic services or amenities may be found. For example, usually Oxford House residents may find a grocery store, pharmacy/chemist, church/synagogue, or bank. Furthermore, residents may easily find health care facilities (e.g., medical or dental care) within their local neighborhood. Less frequently, but still available, Australian compared to U.S. residents seemed more likely to find a public library, movie theatre, post office, or park near their Oxford House.

TABLE 2. Percentage of Neighborhood Amenities and Services Within a Half-Mile of Oxford House

| | OXFORD HOUSES | |
	Australia *(n = 6)*	United States *(n = 55)*
AMENITIES/SERVICES:		
Grocery store	83.3	84.8
Pharmacy/chemist	83.3	77.4
Church/synagogue	83.3	78.8
Bank	100	89.2
Hospital	66.7	73.1
Medical clinic	83.3	82.2
Physician office	100	73.5
Dentist office	83.3	81.5
Public library	83.3	40.4
Movie theatre	66.7	27.8
Post office	100	51.9
Park(s)	100	66.2

Note. U.S. data include all Houses surveyed in Virginia, Illinois, and Hawaii.

DISCUSSION

Studies indicated that Oxford House residents reflect the profile of most other recovering substance abusers (Jason, Davis, Ferrari, & Bishop, 2001), yet living in a community of abstinent others makes their *house* a *home* (Ferrari et al., 2002). Our present study contributes to the line of work profiling the dwelling characteristics (Ferrari et al., 2004) and the community setting of each House (Ferrari et al., 2006). Specifically, the present observation of Oxford Houses from three diverse sections of the United States as well as Australia indicates that these Houses are established in "safe and abstinent settings" where community resources are accessible. From a public health perspective we believe that because residents live in rather similar neighborhoods with many services and amenities their recovery process may be facilitated. Abstinence may be prolonged as individuals acquire skills, services, and resources necessary to control abstinence throughout life (Jason, Olson, Ferrari, & Davis, 2004).

Future Research and Implications

We realize that considerable further study is needed on the Oxford House model and on assessing neighborhood characteristics. For instance, the small sample size of Australian Houses made it impossible to compare them with our U.S. House samples. Future studies should examine larger Houses and ascertain cross-cultural similarities and differences among Houses. In addition, it might have been useful to include other U.S. Houses than just the three states used in the present study. Nevertheless, we believe that our collective body of research will add substantially to an understanding of the role of Oxford House in addiction recovery and provide practical tools that may be generalized to other public health areas. The Oxford House model's emphasis on peer relationships in a cost-effective setting may be useful in the design of other treatment programs desiring to create a "home" atmosphere among participants who live with similar "brothers" or "sisters."

REFERENCES

Cooper, C. (1974). The house as symbol of the self. In J. Lang (Ed.). *Designing for human behavior*. Stroudsburg, PA: Dowden, Hutchinson, & Ross.

Ferrari, J. R., Jason, L. A., Olson, B. D., Davis, M. I., & Alvarez, J. (2002). Sense of community among Oxford House residents recovering from substance abuse: Making a house a home. In A. T. Fisher, C. S. Sonn, & N. J. Bishop (Eds.) *Psychological sense of community: Research, applications, and implications* (pp. 109-122). New York: Kluwer Academic.

Ferrari, J. R., Jason, L. A., Sasser, K., Davis, M. I., & Olson, B. D. (2006). Creating a home to promote recovery: The physical environments of Oxford House. *Journal of Prevention & Intervention in the Community, 31*(1/2), 27-39.

Ferrari, J. R., Jason, L. A., Davis, M. I., Olson, B. D., & Alvarez, J. (2004). Similarities and differences in governance among residents in drug and/or alcohol misuse recovery: Self vs. staff rules and regulations. *Therapeutic Communities, 25*, 185-198.

Jason, L. A., Davis, M. I., Ferrari, J. R., & Bishop, P. (2001) Oxford House: A review of research and implications for substance abuse recovery and community research. *Journal of Drug Education, 31*, 1-27.

Jason, L. A., Ferrari, J. R., Dvorchak, P. A., Groessl, E. J., & Molloy, J. P. (1997). The characteristics of alcoholics in self-help residential treatment settings: A multi-site study of Oxford House. *Alcoholism Treatment Quarterly, 15,* 53-63.

Jason, L. A., Olson, B. D., Ferrari, J. R., & Davis, M. I. (2004). Substance abuse: The need for second order change. *International Journal of Self-help and Self-care, 2,* 91-100.

Jason, L. A., Roberts, K., & Olson, B. D. (2005). Attitudes toward recovery homes and residents: Does proximity make a difference? *Journal of Community Psychology* (in press).

Oxford House, Inc. (1998). *Oxford House Manual.* Silver Spring, MD.

Sigmon, S. T., Whitcomb, S. R., & Snyder, C. R. (2002). Psychological home. In A.T. Fisher, C. S. Sonn, & B. J. Bishop (Eds.), pp. 25-41, *Psychological sense of community: Research, applications, and implications.* New York: Kluwer/Plenum Publications.

Chapter 5:
The Influence of Policy
on the Differential Expansion
of Male and Female Self-Run Recovery Settings

Jordan M. Braciszewski

Wayne State University

Bradley D. Olson
Leonard A. Jason
Joseph R. Ferrari

DePaul University

SUMMARY. The present study used archival data to examine the differential growth among self-governed substance abuse recovery homes for men (N = 443) and women (N = 125). The number of these homes increased dramatically across the U.S. from 1988-1999 when state loan

Address correspondence to: Jordan M. Braciszewski, Wayne State University, Research Group on Homelessness and Poverty, 71 West Warren Avenue, Detroit, MI 48202.

The authors would like to thank the staff at Oxford House, Inc. for providing the data for this study.

The authors appreciate the financial support from the National Institute on Drug Abuse (Grant # DA13231) and the National Institute on Alcohol Abuse and Alcoholism and (Grant # AA12218).

[Haworth co-indexing entry note]: "Chapter 5: The Influence of Policy on the Differential Expansion of Male and Female Self-Run Recovery Settings." Braciszewski, Jordan M. et al. Co-published simultaneously in *Journal of Prevention & Intervention in the Community* (The Haworth Press, Inc.) Vol. 31, No. 1/2, 2006, pp. 51-62; and: *Creating Communities for Addiction Recovery: The Oxford House Model* (ed: Jason et al.) The Haworth Press, Inc., 2006, pp. 51-62. Single or multiple copies of this article are available for a fee from The Haworth Document Delivery Service [1-800-HAWORTH, 9:00 a.m. - 5:00 p.m. (EST). E-mail address: docdelivery@haworthpress.com].

Available online at http://www.haworthpress.com/web/JPIC
doi:10.1300/J005v31n01_05

funds were made available to states and technical assistance was utilized by organizations developing the houses. State loan programs and the utilization of technical assistance, however, had the strongest impact on the expansion of women's houses compared to men's houses. The implications of these findings in relation to the scarcity of recovery options for women are discussed. *[Article copies available for a fee from The Haworth Document Delivery Service: 1-800-HAWORTH. E-mail address: <docdelivery@ haworthpress.com> Website: <http://www.HaworthPress.com> © 2006 by The Haworth Press, Inc. All rights reserved.]*

KEYWORDS. Substance abuse, federal and state policy, mutual-help

The abuse of illicit drugs and alcohol in the United States has produced numerous health problems, including loss of employment, disruptive family relations, increased violence, school failure, suicide, homelessness, and unintended pregnancy (Cartwright, 1999; National Institute on Drug Abuse (NIDA), 2003). Societal costs attributable to substance abuse have reached over $500 billion a year in the U.S., including services for substance abuse treatment and prevention and other healthcare and medical programs. In addition, these figures also account for lost earnings due to illness and premature death and losses associated with criminal activity and substance abuse-related accidents (Horgan, Skwara, Strickler, Andersen, & Stein, 2001).

Consequently, there is an increased need for cost-effective substance abuse treatment modalities that serve diverse populations (see d'Arlach, Curtis, Ferrari, Olson, & Jason, 2005; Ferrari, Jason, Olson, Davis, & Alvarez, 2002; Jason, Olson, Ferrari, & Davis, 2003). For most individuals, treatment and recovery work best in a community-centered system of numerous services designed to ensure a variety of support for recovery (Center for Substance Abuse Treatment, 1993).

Oxford House is one potential option for individuals seeking drug-free housing that meets these needs. Founded in 1975, the Oxford House model illustrates a community-based approach toward substance abstinence. Unlike traditional residential care where trained professionals mandate and enforce rules and policies and set a maximum length of stay, Oxford House offers residential communities without a set length of stay and without the involvement of professional treatment staff (Oxford House Manual, 1988). The model offers a supportive, democratic, self-help setting where individuals recovering from alcohol and drug addiction work together to develop long-term abstinence skills (Jason et al., 2003; Jason, Ferrari, Dvorchak, Groessl, & Molloy, 1997). Oxford House residents receive intensive 12-step support from peers, develop the rules and structure and, therefore, are potentially more likely to become invested in the recovery setting (Ferrari, Jason, Olson, Davis, & Alvarez, 2003).

The initial expansion of Oxford Houses occurred in part due to grassroots efforts (e.g., cohabitants in an existing Oxford House providing loan funds to others in recovery to open a new house). From 1975 to 1988, 15 Oxford Houses (all male) were developed and maintained through these grassroots expansion methods. In the hopes of generating more Oxford House-like settings, the *Anti-Drug Abuse Act* of 1988 mandated that all states make revolving loan funds available to open up self-run recovery homes. States that utilized these funds for technical assistance typically hired outreach workers to open and monitor the new houses (Oxford House Manual, 1988). Further, outreach workers informed local treatment facilities of existing and planned houses, and secured initial amenities for the residents.

However, all states were not required to offer loan funds when the Anti-Drug Abuse Act was revised in 1999. The majority of states with established outreach workers continued to maintain their loan funds. In the years following 1999, states that had not utilized technical assistance (e.g., hired outreach workers) eliminated the availability of their loan funds (J. P. Molloy, personal communication, February 23, 2004). The availability of this loan fund and the hiring of outreach workers within utilization states had dramatically increased the number of Oxford Houses opened across the country. Jason, Braciszewski, Olson, and Ferrari (2005) found, for instance, that states utilizing technical assistance experienced greater Oxford House growth when compared to states that had not utilized this assistance. Since only the total number of houses affected by the policy was examined, it is unclear whether this policy intervention differentially affected the growth of male versus female houses.

There are a number of reasons to investigate potential gender effects this policy may have had on the opening of Oxford Houses across the country. Research indicates for instance that the gender gap in substance use has narrowed in recent years (NIDA, 2003; Substance Abuse and Mental Health Services Administration (SAMHSA), 1999a; 2000; 2003). In the late 1970s to the early 1990s, about 4% of women used either alcohol or illicit drugs daily (Abelson, 1977; SAMHSA, 1996), while that figure rose to 8% by the late 1990s (SAMHSA, 1999b). Research has also demonstrated that, after initial use, women may become addicted to drugs and alcohol in a shorter time period than men (Alvarez, Olson, Jason, Davis, & Ferrari, 2004; Davis, Carpenter, Malte, Carney, Chambers, & Saxon, 2002; Wechsberg, Craddock, & Hubbard, 1998).

The increase in the number of women with substance abuse problems has not been accompanied by an equivalent increase in treatment availability (see d'Arlach et al., in press). SAMHSA (1997) research indicates that only 30% of women who required substance abuse treatment actually received it. Some researchers suggest that women are also less likely than men to seek treatment due to the lack of drug-free housing, long waiting lists within treatment facilities, and the ability to pay for residential treatment (Coletti, 1998; d'Arlach et al., in press; Dvorchak, Grams, Tate, & Jason, 1995; Moras, 1998; Olson, Curtis, Jason, Ferrari, Horin, Davis et al., 2003). Given the individual and social problems associated with addiction (Fields, 1988), it seems crucial to identify factors that affect the development and growth of gender-sensitive and empowering recovery models that serve both women and men.

Due to the self-liberating nature of the Oxford House model, these types of recovery homes may be an aftercare treatment modality that is likely to address these gender-specific issues (Dvorchak et al., 1995). Over the past 29 years, Oxford Houses have grown to over 1,000 in the U.S. with a 3:1 ratio of men's to women's houses (J. P. Molloy, personal communication, March 2004). While this ratio is typical of other substance abuse treatment programs, tracing the expansion of this model may help explain this disparity. The grassroots model that provided the impetus for the initial growth of Oxford Houses, for instance, may have led members of existing houses to open future houses of the same gender (e.g., the early foundation of 15 male houses encouraging the early opening of more male houses). These trends are perhaps less likely to occur when houses are opened through the utilization of federal and state technical assistance that mandate gender-balanced settings (i.e., more women's houses).

The present study investigated the potential impact of federal policy and technical assistance on the development and expansion of men and women's self-run recovery homes known as Oxford Houses. Specifically, we hypothesized that women's houses expanded more rapidly in states that utilized technical assistance. In contrast, in states that did not utilize technical assistance or dropped the loan fund in 1999, we expected a greater decline among women's compared to men's houses. Because the initial grassroots efforts and subsequent openings were predominately male, the expansion of male houses is more likely to remain consistent and stable.

METHOD

Setting Information

Archival data were obtained from Oxford House, Inc. on homes opened between 1988 and 2002 (M. Brown, personal communication, September 2003). Data included the gender of the house, the date when a house was opened, and whether each house was opened in a state that hired outreach workers to provide technical assistance. State-level data were collected assessing the periods in which each state possessed the revolving loan fund and/or implemented technical assistance to open the houses.

Overall, the study included 568 Oxford Houses[1] (443 male, 125 female) that were opened between 1988 and July 2002 and remained opened throughout this period. Of these houses, 448 (79%) were opened between 1988 and 1999 (Time 1) when states were mandated by the Anti-Drug Abuse Act to provide the revolving loan fund. An additional 120 Oxford Houses (21%) were opened between 2000 and July 2002 (Time 2) after the loan mandate was discontinued.

Of the 568 houses opened, 507 (89%) were developed in states that employed at least one outreach worker who provided technical assistance. Of the 507 houses opened with the utilization of technical assistance, 394 houses (78%) were men's houses and 113 (22%) were women's houses.

Statistical Analyses

The primary analysis involved the examination of technical assistance and its differential impact on the gender of houses being opened across the two time periods. However, it was important to first investigate potential base-rate differences in men and women's houses using chi-square and binomial non-parametric analyses. The effect of technical assistance on the opening of Oxford Houses across the country was also explored, while controlling for the difference in the number of states that utilized this assistance. We expected that technical assistance would have a positive impact on the rate of all houses opened, but particularly assist in the expansion of women's houses.

RESULTS

Men's and Women's Houses

To examine potential base-rate differences between men (N = 443) and women's (N = 125) houses nationally, non-parametric techniques were used. *Chi-square tests* indicated a significant gender difference in the opening of houses, $\chi^2(1, N = 568) = 178.035$, $p < .001$, where 78% of all openings were male houses. However, a more conservative approach that accounts for these disparities in male and female houses is to use the binomial non-parametric test, which permitted the comparison of observed (number of actual men and women's Oxford Houses) and expected proportional indices. The observed proportion of male houses ($\pi = .78$, or 443/568) again was found to be significantly greater than the expected proportion ($\pi = .66$), $z = 6.03$, $p < .001$. This expected proportion was derived from NIDA (2003) and SAMHSA (2003) data indicating that approximately 66% of the substance abusing population is male. Therefore, regardless of the disparity in the number of men and women's houses opened, the proportion of men's houses opened to the total number of houses opened was significantly greater than the expected proportion of .66.

Utilization of Technical Assistance

As stated earlier, 507 of the 568 houses (89%) were opened in states utilizing technical assistance. Due to the categorical nature of the data, *chi-square* tests were used for the analysis. Results indicated that significantly more houses were opened in states utilizing this assistance compared to states that did not use this assistance, $\chi^2(1, N = 568) = 350.204$, $p < .001$. Of the 26 states in the present study, however, only 12 states utilized outreach workers to develop and expand house growth. In order to statistically confirm the behavioral analyses that more houses were opened in utilization states (Jason et al., 2004), the 26 states were matched by population and income using independent samples *t-tests* to account for any socio-economic differences that might be related to house expansion. No significant differences were found on state population and median income among the matched states, $t(17) = -.82$, $p =$

.424 and $t(24) = 1.549$, $p = .135$, allowing us to make the necessary statistical comparisons. Results indicated that houses opened in states employing outreach workers to provide technical assistance ($\pi = .89$, or 507/568) opened significantly more houses than states that did not utilize this assistance ($\pi = .11$, or 61/568), $z = 20.65$, $p < .000$.

Changes in National Policy

It was also necessary to examine trends in house expansion associated with national policy changes. In 1999, states were no longer mandated to provide self-run recovery home loan funds. We proposed that the utilization of technical assistance positively affected the opening of women's Oxford Houses more than men's houses from 1999 to 2002. Furthermore, we projected that the lack of technical assistance and termination of the state revolving loan fund would have a negative effect on the expansion of women's but not men's homes. Thus it was logical to assume that 1999 represented the time period when house expansion was most likely to be affected by policy utilization.

The primary analyses were to examine the impact of state utilization of technical assistance on the opening of houses by gender across time using *chi-square* analyses. The disparity in the number of years in each time period (Time 1, $n = 11$; and Time 2, $n = 2.5$) was controlled by standardizing the number of houses opened in Time 2. This process was achieved by multiplying the number of houses in Time 2 by 4.4 (the relative difference between the 2.5 years represented by Time 2 and the 11 years represented by Time 1). Results indicated that the number of female houses opened across the two time periods significantly increased in states that had utilized technical assistance, $\chi^2(1, N = 221) = 14.7$, $p = .0001$, and had a directional decrease in states that had not utilized technical assistance, $\chi^2(1, N = 15) = 3.27$, $p = .07$ (see Figure 1). In contrast, the number of male houses opened across the two time periods increased slightly regardless of whether the houses were opened in states that had not utilized technical assistance, $\chi^2(1, N = 86) = 1.16$, $p = .28$, or those that had utilized technical assistance, $\chi^2(1, N = 656) = .74$, $p = .39$.

DISCUSSION

The present findings suggest that a major influence on the expansion of Oxford Houses was the utilization of state loan funds to hire outreach

FIGURE 1. Number of Oxford Houses Opened Across Time by Technical Assistance and Gender (standardized for number of years).

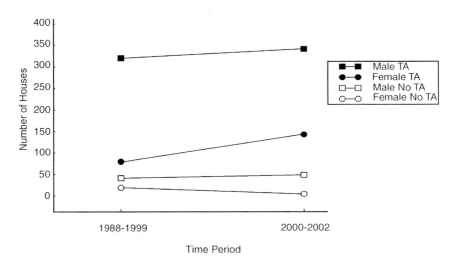

workers to both open and monitor new houses. While the relative shortage of Oxford Houses for women is consistent with the current state of recovery and treatment options for women across the country (NIDA, 2003), the disparity was somewhat reduced by state policy assistance geared toward the expansion of self-run recovery homes. However, a significant gender gap in substance abuse recovery options still remains. The strategic placement of federal and state resources may influence the development and expansion of community-based resources in the form of self-run recovery homes. While raw data for the number of houses suggest this is true for the opening of men's houses over time (and having such aid fostered the growth of more men's houses when compared to not having outreach workers), these resources had a more substantial positive influence on the opening of women's homes (and harmed them more once the loan fund was no longer available).

Although the utilization of technical assistance helped to open a greater number of male houses, this aid seemed to more substantially impact the relative opening of women's Oxford Houses for several reasons. The initial grassroots efforts in establishing the model for recovery and the opening of Oxford Houses were conducted primarily by men in recovery. Because the grassroots expansion of houses occurred through existing networks (e.g., several residents of an established house moving into a new house until it is stable), the composition of houses spread through these efforts would more likely reflect the gender of the original, surrounding houses. Perhaps if the initial houses were women's houses, a bias toward the opening of women's houses may have existed.

In addition, once loan funds were in place within states and outreach workers were hired, provisions may have been in place that encouraged a greater balance of men and women's houses. Perhaps of most consequence is that while raw data indicate that more male houses have been opened over the years, proportional indices clearly demonstrate that the impact on the expansion of women's homes has been more substantial than when assistance has not been utilized or available. Because of federal regulations for state-supported funds, equal opportunity laws may more likely lead to the hiring of an equivalent number of male and female outreach workers to develop Oxford Houses within the state. Subsequently, female workers may have opened more women's houses and male outreach workers opened men's houses.

Overall, the present study suggests that federal and state resources (in the form of loan funds and the provision of outreach workers) were effective in increasing the number of Oxford Houses in those states that actualized these resources. There exists a goal to find more gender-sensitive forms of substance abuse treatment modalities. Many components of Oxford House may be seen as gender-sensitive. For instance, women are allowed the freedom to design their own recovery plans to meet their specific needs, empowering them with a more flexible, autonomous recovery experience (Dvorchak et al., 1995). Greater self-governance may also provide increased control over their lives and more supportive relationships among other women residents. Such a high sense of community may impart active coping and interpersonal skills that are likely to decrease feelings of hopelessness and other emotions associated with depression/learned helplessness—often found in women recovering from or experiencing substance abuse problems (Luthar & Walsh, 1995; Olson et al., 2003; Osgood & Manetta, 2000).

It is possible to infer that while the initial grassroots efforts of the Oxford House movement alone may have not been a particularly large catalyst for the development of women's houses, it was shown that public policy and the utilization of that policy may have a significant impact on the presence of more recovery opportunities for women. It remains necessary for researchers to explore varied methods of opening houses. Because self-run recovery homes are likely to have the potential to offer a more gender-sensitive form of treatment, the greater expansion of such homes may provide women with better opportunities to initiate recovery earlier and more effectively. Enhanced accessibility of state funds and the use of outreach workers seem to be of prime importance to the growth of self-run homes such as Oxford House, offering a more context- and culture-specific method of recovery. It is important that research and public policy explore this question further, as this study has shown that even with extensive resources to open recovery homes for women, the gender gap, represented by total number of houses opened, continues to be vast. Future research should examine state-level variables that can contribute to the promotion of these loan funds and subsequent assistance in the development of self-run recovery homes.

NOTE

1. Although the sample size in the current study is $n = 568$, there is in 2004 over 1,000 houses. This is partly due to data collection ending in mid-2002 and partly due to several states within inconsistent utilization of technical assistance that were excluded from the study.

REFERENCES

Abelson, H. I., Fishburne, P. M., & Crisin, I. (1977). *National Survey on Drug Abuse, Vol. 1: Main Findings.* National Institute on Drug Abuse: Rockville, MD.

Alvarez, J., Olson, B. D., Jason, L. A., Davis, M. I., & Ferrari, J. R. (2004). Heterogeneity among Latinas and Latinos in substance abuse treatment: Findings from a national database. *Journal of Substance Abuse Treatment.*

Cartwright, W. S. (1999). Costs of drug abuse to society. *The Journal of Mental Health Policy and Economics, 2,* 133-134.

Center for Substance Abuse Treatment. (1993). *Screening for infectious diseases among substance abusers* (Treatment improvement protocol (TIP) series 6). DHHS Pub. No. SMA 93-2048. Rockville, MD: U.S. Dept. of Health and Human Services.

Coletti, S. D. (1998). Service provider/Treatment access issues. In C. L. Wetherington & A. B. Roman (Eds.), *Drug addiction research and the health of women: Executive summary* (pp. 58-66). National Institute on Drug Abuse; NIH Publication No. 98-4289.

d'Arlach, L., Curtis, C. E., Ferrari, J. R., Olson, B. D., & Jason, L. A. (2005). Substance-abusing women and their children: A cost-effective treatment option. *Journal of Social Work Practice in the Addictions,* in press.

Davis, M., Carpenter, K. M., Malte, C. A., Carney, M., Chambers, S., & Saxon, A. (2002). Women in addictions treatment: Comparing VA and community samples. *Journal of Substance Abuse Treatment, 23,* 41-48.

Dvorchak, P. A., Grams, G., Tate, L., & Jason, L. A. (1995). Pregnant and postpartum women in recovery: Barriers to treatment and the role of Oxford House in the continuation of care. *Alcoholism Treatment Quarterly, 13,* 97-107.

Ferrari, J. R., Jason, L. A., Olson, B., Davis, M., & Alvarez, J. (2002). Sense of community among Oxford House residents recovering from substance abuse. In A. T. Fisher, C. C. Sonn, & B. J. Bishop (Eds.), *Psychological Sense of Community: Research, Applications, and Implications* (pp. 109-122). New York: Kluwer/Plenum.

Ferrari, J. R., Jason, L. A., Olson, B., Davis, M., & Alvarez, J. (2004). Assessing similarities and differences in governance among residential recovery programs: Self versus staff rules and regulations. *Therapeutic Communities: The International Journal for Therapeutic and Supportive Organizations, 25,* 185-198..

Fields, R. (1988). *Drugs in perspective* (3rd ed.). Boston, MA: McGraw-Hill.

Horgan, C., Skwara, K. C., Strickler, G., Andersen, L., & Stein, J. (Ed.). (2001). *Substance Abuse: The Nation's Number One Health Problem.* Princeton, NJ: Robert Wood Johnson Foundation.

Jason, L. A., Braciszewski, J. M., Olson, B. D., & Ferrari, J. R. (2005). Increasing the number of mutual help recovery homes for substance abusers: Effects of government policy and funding assistance. *Behavioral and Social Issues, 14,* 70-78.

Jason, L. A., Ferrari, J. R., Dvorchak, P. A., Groessl, E. J., & Malloy, J. P. (1997). The characteristics of alcoholics in self-help residential treatment settings: A multi-site study of Oxford House. *Alcoholism Treatment Quarterly, 15,* 53-63.

Jason, L. A., Olson, B. D., Ferrari, J. R., & Davis, M. I. (2003). Substance abuse: The need for second-order change. *International Journal of Self Help and Self Care, 2,* 91-109.

Luthar, S. S., & Walsh, K. G. (1995). Treatment needs of drug-addicted mothers. *Journal of Substance Abuse Treatment, 12,* 341-348.

Moras, K. (1998). Psychosocial and behavioral treatments for women. In C. L. Wetherington & A. B. Roman (Eds.), *Drug addiction research and the health of women: Executive summary* (pp. 49-52). National Institute on Drug Abuse: NIH Publication No. 98-4289.

National Institute on Drug Abuse. (2003). *Epidemiologic Trends in Drug Abuse* (NIH Publication No. 04-5364A). Bethesda, MD: National Institutes of Health.

Olson, B. D., Curtis, C. E., Jason, L. A., Ferrari, J. R., Horin, E. V. et al. (2003). Physical and sexual trauma, psychiatric symptoms, and sense of community among women in recovery: Toward a new model of shelter aftercare. *Journal of Prevention & Intervention in the Community, 26,* 67-80.

Osgood, N. J., & Manetta, A. A. (2000). Abuse and suicidal issues in older women. *Journal of Death and Dying, 42,* 71-81.

Oxford House, Inc. (1988). *Oxford House Manual.* Silver Spring, MD.

Substance Abuse and Mental Health Services Administration. (1996). *National Household Survey on Drug Abuse: Main findings 1994* (DHHS Publication No. SMA 96-3085). Rockville, MD: Office of Applied Studies.

Substance Abuse and Mental Health Services Administration. (1997). *Substance use among women in the United States, 1997* (DHHS Publication No. SMA 97-3162). Rockville, MD: Office of Applied Studies.

Substance Abuse and Mental Health Services Administration. (1999a). *Results from the 1997 National Household Survey on Drug Abuse: Main Findings* (DHHS Pub. No. SMA 99-3295). Rockville, MD: Office of Applied Studies.

Substance Abuse and Mental Health Services Administration. (1999b). *Summary of findings from the 1998 National Household Survey on Drug Abuse* (DHHS Publication No. SMA 99-3328). Rockville, MD: Office of Applied Studies.

Substance Abuse and Mental Health Services Administration. (2000). *Results from the 1998 National Household Survey on Drug Abuse: Main Findings* (DHHS Pub. No. SMA 00-3381). Rockville, MD: Office of Applied Studies.

Substance Abuse and Mental Health Services Administration. (2003). *Results from the 2002 National Survey on Drug Use and Health: National Findings* (DHHS Publication No. SMA 03-3836). Rockville, MD: Office of Applied Studies.

Wechsberg, W. M., Craddock, S. G., & Hubbard, R. L. (1998). How are women who enter substance abuse treatment different than men? A gender comparison from the Drug Abuse Treatment Outcome Study. *Drugs & Society, 13,* 97-115.

Chapter 6:
Economic Costs of Oxford House Inpatient Treatment and Incarceration: A Preliminary Report

Bradley D. Olson
Judah J. Viola
Leonard A. Jason

DePaul University

Margaret I. Davis

Dickinson College

Joseph R. Ferrari
Olga Rabin-Belyaev

DePaul University

SUMMARY. The Oxford House model for substance abuse recovery has potential economic advantages associated with the low cost of open-

Address correspondence to: Bradley D. Olson, DePaul University, Center for Community Research, 990 West Fullerton Avenue, Suite 3100, Chicago, IL 60614-2458.

The authors appreciate the financial support from the National Institute on Drug Abuse (Grant # DA13231) and the National Institute on Alcohol Abuse and Alcoholism (Grant # AA12218).

[Haworth co-indexing entry note]: "Chapter 6: Economic Costs of Oxford House Inpatient Treatment and Incarceration: A Preliminary Report." Olson, Bradley D. et al. Co-published simultaneously in *Journal of Prevention & Intervention in the Community* (The Haworth Press, Inc.) Vol. 31, No. 1/2, 2006, pp. 63-72; and: *Creating Communities for Addiction Recovery: The Oxford House Model* (ed: Jason et al.) The Haworth Press, Inc., 2006, pp. 63-72. Single or multiple copies of this article are available for a fee from The Haworth Document Delivery Service [1-800- HAWORTH, 9:00 a.m. - 5:00 p.m. (EST). E-mail address: docdelivery@haworthpress.com].

Available online at http://www.haworthpress.com/web/JPIC
doi:10.1300/J005v31n01_06

ing up and maintaining the settings. In the present study, annual program costs per person were estimated for Oxford House based on federal loan information and data collected from Oxford House Inc. In addition, annual treatment and incarceration costs were approximated based on participant data prior to Oxford House residence in conjunction with normative costs for these settings. Societal costs associated with the Oxford House program were relatively low, whereas estimated costs associated with inpatient and incarceration history were high. The implications of these findings are discussed. *[Article copies available for a fee from The Haworth Document Delivery Service: 1-800-HAWORTH. E-mail address: <docdelivery@ haworthpress.com> Website: <http://www.HaworthPress. com> © 2006 by The Haworth Press, Inc. All rights reserved.]*

KEYWORDS. Economic, cost, substance abuse, mutual-help, Oxford House

A central concern associated with providing effective social services involves locating the best and most comprehensive forms of therapeutic support within the realistic confines of public and private cost (Drummond, O'Brien, Stoddart, & Torrance, 1997). Addiction-related services, in particular, are strongly dependent on such cost considerations (Cartwright, 2000; French, Salomé, Sindelar, & Mclellan, 2002; Yates, 1994; Zarkin, 1998). The national monetary figures associated with substance abuse are in the hundreds of billions of dollars annually. They include treatment, legal and incarceration costs; property damage; victim harm; employment attrition and loss of productivity; and medical care for sexually transmitted diseases, alcohol-induced cirrhosis, fetal alcohol syndrome, cardiovascular disease, and a variety of cancers (NIDA, 1998; Ponitz, Olson, Jason, Davis, & Ferrari, 2006; Zarkin; Robert Wood Johnson Foundation, 1999). Treatment alone has the potential to significantly decrease these societal costs. However, the economic benefits to be gained through treatment can be maximized by retaining program efficacy while reducing base program costs.

The most commonly chosen approach in the U.S. to lowering taxpayer investment associated with program costs has been to reduce the duration of services (Jason, Olson, Ferrari, & Davis, 2004). The *brief intervention*, for instance, attempts to target problematic use early through an intense intervention often occurring within a single session (Zweben & Fleming, 1999). The *recovery management checkups* model is another innovative method to increase long-term maintenance and monitoring through brief visits following traditional (or shortened) treatment stays (Dennis, Scott, & Funk, 2003). While distinct advantages exist in utilizing these brief methods, the commonly severe and chronic nature of substance abuse dependence more often than not requires them to be used in conjunction with more comprehensive and therefore more costly services, thus curbing their ultimate economic value.

Duration of services is often associated with higher program costs, yet also more successful forms of recovery (Yates, 1994). Length of time within a therapeutic community, for instance, has been associated with more effective recovery outcomes (see Jason et al., 2004). The therapeutic community, one of the most comprehensive and therefore most costly forms of care for substance abuse addiction, has nevertheless demonstrated impressive overall cost-effectiveness estimates (French, Sacks, DeLeon, Staines, & McKendrick, 1999). Cost-benefit ratios can increase further if services are provided that are of equivalent duration as the therapeutic community and similar in other benefits but implemented at lower costs.

One recovery option that has extended the duration of support and requires little to no taxpayer investment is the mutual-help group, such as Alcoholics Anonymous (AA) (McCrady & Miller, 1993). Twelve-step programs require little other operational costs than gathering expenses (e.g., photocopying, refreshments), all donated by members themselves. Despite the low societal program costs, little research has been attempted to obtain precise cost effectiveness estimates associated with AA attendance. Such research may be uncommon because social scientists perceive the difficulties associated with studying a group that values self-protection from external influences, and is not likely to be interested in policy changes should economic research suggest them. Therefore, while 12-step programs have, and likely will always, play a significant role in low-cost recovery, challenges will continue to exist for gaining in-depth economic understanding and engaging in subsequent policy strategies with this recovery option.

The Oxford House model of mutual-help recovery homes possesses many advantages of the above programs: the comprehensive and long-term support of the therapeutic community, the reduced tax-burden element of AA, and yet, nevertheless has demonstrated an openness to state and federal involvement. Oxford Houses are democratic, self-run homes based on the 12-step model, functioning without professional staff. The primary operational costs are associated with rent paid by the residents (Jason et al., 1997). The opening and expansion of the model furthermore has led to approximately 1000 houses in the United States, and also requires minimal costs, often having been developed through funds provided by existing houses. Oxford House has also grown through federal/state initiatives with revolving loan funds distributed to states according to the Federal Anti-Drug Abuse Act of 1988. Whereas these policy initiatives cost more in tax-payer funds than the grassroots forms of expansion, the amounts are still minimal compared to traditional interventions. The majority of such costs are invested in the allocation of furniture, security deposit/down payment of rent and in the hiring of outreach workers to set up and initially stabilize a collection of houses (Braciszewski, Olson, Jason, & Ferrari, 2006; Jason, Braciszewski, Olson, & Ferrari, 2005; Molloy, 1993).

While the ideal form of research in this area is represented by prospective economic evaluations investigating the relationship of cost to benefit, it is important to establish the societal cost of programs like Oxford House. In the present study, we attempt to establish the annual, per person estimates of societal program costs associated with Oxford House (i.e., the opening and maintaining of houses). We also derive conservative estimates of societal inpatient treatment costs and incarceration costs based on national data of individuals prior to entering Oxford House and ranges of normative costs associated with these settings (i.e., inpatient treatment, jail, and prison). Data were obtained from 90-day data on the inpatient treatment and incarceration history of residents prior to entering Oxford House.

METHOD

Societal Oxford House Program Costs. To obtain annual, per person societal cost estimates associated with the opening and maintenance of an Oxford House, loan fund information was obtained and verified from several state and federal sources (e.g., SAMSHA) in addition to Oxford House Inc. (Molloy, personal communication, February 2004). Additional estimates were obtained from various development grants and contracts funded to open Oxford Houses (e.g., Veterans Affairs funding). Estimates from several of the sources include operational costs for larger organizations, and while these costs are rarely necessary for the successful opening of Oxford Houses, the inclusion of these estimates contributes to the conservative goals of this analysis. The base figures to open an Oxford House, as described, generally include funds for security deposit, first month's rent, furniture and amenities, and, in broader state-wide efforts, the hiring of outreach workers (Molloy, 1993). The present system of revolving loan funds are repaid by house residents, but again are nevertheless included in the estimates to contribute to the conservative approach. Rent beyond one month, however, which is provided by the residents, cannot be interpreted as tax-base related costs (i.e., societal costs), and therefore are not included within the estimates.

Societal Inpatient Treatment and Incarceration Program Costs. For cost estimates of societal inpatient and incarceration costs, information was used from a national dataset of Oxford House residents. The total dataset was of 900 participants from over 200 houses, and collected from five primary regions within the U.S., including Washington/Oregon, Texas, Illinois, Pennsylvania/New Jersey, and the Carolinas. The majority of participants completed the baseline battery in their Oxford Houses and a minority filled out the inventories at an Oxford House convention. Significant differences by house, region, or method of collection were not found. Participants had been given $15 for their participation.

The 90-day *Timeline Follow-back* measure (Carter-Sobell, Agrawal, Sobell, Leo, Young, Cunningham, & Simco, 2003) provided data on past inpatient treatment history and incarceration time of participants, and its use is consistent with that of the *Addiction Severity Index* to obtain sample-derived societal costs in prior economic studies (French et al., 2002). While the database consisted of information on a sample of 900, 269 of these participants provided the investigators at least 30-90 days of data available on their incarceration and inpatient treatment experiences prior to entering the Oxford House. Only the data from this sample of 269 participants was included in the present analyses, providing an average of 63.9 days (range 30-90) of pre-Oxford House data. The average number of inpatient treatment days for this residence-time differentiated sample was 17 days (range: 0 to 90 days), 3.70 days for jail (range 0 to 75), and 1.87 days for prison (range: 0 to 90 days).

Additional necessary information for estimates required normative figures reflecting average societal costs (facility and operational) for inpatient treatment, jail, and prison, making them comparable to the societal program cost estimates of Oxford House. This data was gathered from archival public sources (e.g., U.S. Department of Justice, 2003). Based on these estimates, costs were extrapolated for all 269 participants. Number of days for inpatient treatment, jail, and prison were transformed into single day figures and then annualized. The financial estimates of treatment and incarceration costs were finally adjusted for inflation at a conservative 3% rate of growth from the year reported in the source to 2004 (Levy, 1995).

RESULTS

Estimates of annual per person costs first required house costs, which ranged from $4,000 to $22,000 per Oxford House. The higher end of the range reflects the attempt to remain conservative because the modal cost is more likely to reflect the lower end of the range (i.e., $4,000). Based on a national average of seven residents per house, the annual estimates per person ranged from $571.43 to $3,142.86, the latter figure reflecting the upper end of larger statewide-scale initiatives.

Societal inpatient treatment costs were based on the Oxford House sample, estimates from prior research sources (French, Salomé, Sindelar, & Mclellan, 2002), and subsequent adjustments for inflation increases. Average yearly approximations of societal costs of *inpatient care* for this sample ranged from $3,929.57 (French, Salomé, & Carney, 2002) to $16,964.58 (Schinka, Francis, Hughes, LaLone, & Flynn, 1998).

To obtain final incarceration costs, jail, and prison costs were combined into a single set of estimates. A collection of normative jail costs were first located, and it was evident that the range of figures in the pool were restricted enough to choose one annual, per person, median figure of $17,635 (U.S. Department of Justice, 2003). This jail cost, was averaged with both the lower and higher prison estimates. Because jail costs are consistently lower than prison costs, this approach provided a more conservative overall incarceration estimate. The annual prison cost estimates per inmate ranged from $22,344 (Drug Policy Alliance Ohio, 2002) to $62,927 (Rosten, 2003). Averaging the jail and prison figures, the annual societal program *incarceration* cost estimate per participant ranged from $19,989 to $40,281.

DISCUSSION

In general, data suggest that low annual, per person costs are involved in the opening and maintaining of an Oxford House. Findings from the present study also suggest that annual, per person inpatient treatment and incarceration costs derived from a pre-Oxford House sample are high. The findings presented are preliminary, despite the conservative approach taken throughout the estimation process. There are substantial limits to taking a retrospective approach when conducting economic analyses, and the procedures are no substitute for prospective economic investigations designed to assess cost-effectiveness using measures explicitly created for this purpose (e.g., French et al., 2002).

One advantage of this study is that it represents a first effort to estimate Oxford House costs, in addition to inpatient treatment and incarceration costs based on a relatively large sample of individuals who naturally choose to reside in an Oxford House. Past studies have suggested that the severity and chronic nature of drug use and crime among Oxford House residents are comparable to most treatment samples in the U.S. (Jason et al., 2001; Olson, Jason, Davis, Alvarez, & Ferrari, 2003). Nevertheless, until there is a substantial body of literature demonstrating the comparability of these populations, the use of sample-specific derivations is the most prudent approach to approximate these costs.

As stated above, the present analysis investigated societal program *costs*–not the *cost and benefits* derived from the Oxford House or any other program. Past economic studies in the substance abuse arena that have investigated *benefits* have shown substantial societal savings from a variety of treatment forms (French et al., 1999; Yates, 1994; Zarkin, 1998). Past studies using other treatment modalities have ranged from societal savings of one dollar for every dollar invested in treatment to $18 dollars for every dollar invested (see Salomé, French, Scott, Foss, & Dennis, 2003). A combined examination of cost and benefits is a sensible next step for future Oxford House research. Moreover, comprehensive investigations are needed that examine traditional benefits (e.g., reductions in substance use/crime, and increases in employment) and less traditional benefits (e.g., reductions in victimization from crime, incidence of fetal alcohol syndrome).

There exists a general need to better understand the high costs of inpatient treatment and incarceration, and to investigate a variety of strategies that have the potential to reduce the societal burden. Oxford House can be utilized in conjunction with other recovery options within a continuum of care, as a diversion opportunity for offenders or community-based transition for ex-offenders (Olson et al., 2003). Much of the societal potential of Oxford House in these areas and others is expanded through its openness to federal and state policy involvement (Braciszewski et al., 2006; Jason et al., 2005). More rigorous and comprehensive economic investigations of such community-based options will allow investigators and public policy officials to better understand the possible role of self-run recovery homes within a more comprehensive and integrated substance abuse treatment system.

REFERENCES

Alexandre, P. K., Roebuck, M. C., French, M. T., Barry, M. (2003). The cost of residential addiction treatment in public housing. *Journal of Substance Abuse Treatment 24(4)*, 285-290.

Braciszewski, J. M., Olson, B. D., Jason, L. A., & Ferrari, J. R. (2006). The influence of policy on the differential expansion of male and female self-run recovery settings. *Journal of Prevention & Intervention in the Community*, 31 (1/2), 51-62.

Carbonari, J. P. & DiClemente, C. C. (2000). Using transtheoretical model profiles to differentiate levels of alcohol abstinence success. *Journal of Consulting & Clinical Psychology*. *68(5)*, 810-817.

Carter Sobell, L., Agrawal, S., Sobell, M. B., Leo, G. I., Young, L. J., Cunningham, J. A., & Simco, E. R. (2003). Comparison of a Quick Drinking Screen with the Timeline Follow-back for Individuals with Alcohol Problems. *Journal of Studies on Alcohol*, *64(6)*, 858-861.

Cartwright, W. S. (2000). Cost-benefit analysis of drug treatment services: Review of the literature. *The Journal of Mental Health Policy and Economics*, *3*, 11-26.

d'Arlach, L., Curtis, C. E., Ferrari, J. R., Olson, B. D., & Jason, L. A. (2005). Substance-abusing women and their children: A cost-effective treatment option. *Journal of Social Work Practice in the Addictions*.

Dennis, M., Scott, C. K., & Funk, R. (2003). An experimental evaluation of recovery management checkups (RMC) for people with chronic substance use disorders. *Evaluation and Program Planning*, *26*, 339-352.

Drug Policy Alliance; Ohio (2002). Report Compares Cost of Community Corrections to Prison: Community Based Treatment Less Expensive, May Be More Effective.

Drummond, M. F., O'Brien, B., Stoddart, G. L., & Torrance, G. W. (1997). Methods for the economic evaluation of health care programmes. New York: Oxford University Press.

French, M. T., Mauskopf, J. A., Teague, J. L., & Roland, J. (1996). Estimating the dollar value of health outcomes from drug abuse interventions. *Medical Care, 34 (9)*, 890-910.

French, M. T., Rajkummer, A. S. (1997). Drug abuse, crime costs and the economic benefits of treatment. *Journal of Quantitative Criminology 13(3)*, 291-323.

French, M. T., Salomé, H. J., Sindelar, J. L., & Mclellan, A. T. (2002). Benefit-Cost Analysis of Addiction Treatment, Methodological Guidelines and Empirical Application Using the DATCAP and ASI. *Health Services Research, 37(2)*, 433-455.

French, M. T., Zarkin, G. A., Hubbard, R. L., & Rachal, J. V. (1991). The impact of time in treatment on the employment and earnings of drug abusers. *American Journal of Public Health, 81 (7)*, 904-907.

French, M. T., Sacks, S., DeLeon, G., Staines, G., & McKendrick, K. (1999). Modified therapeutic community for mentally ill chemical abusers: Outcomes and costs. *Evaluation and the Health Professions, 22*, 60-85.

French, M. T., Salomé, H. J., & Carney, M. (2002). Using the DATCAP and ASI to estimate the costs and benefits of residential addiction treatment in the state of Washington. *Social Science & Medicine, 55(12)*, 2267-2282.

Jason, L. A., Olson, B. D., Ferrari, J. R., & Davis, M. I. (2004). Substance abuse: The need for second-order change. *International Journal of Self Help & Self Care, 2(2),* 91-109.

Jason, L. A., Ferrari, J. R., Smith, B., Marsh, P. Dvorchak, P. A., Groessl et al. (1997). An exploratory study of male recovering substance abusers living in a self-help, self-governed setting. *Journal of Mental Health Administration, 24,* 332-339.

Jason, L. A., Pechota, M. E., Bowden, B. S., Lahmar, K., Pokorny, S., Bishop, P., Quintana, E., Sangerman, C., Salina, D., Taylor, S., Lesondak, L., & Grams, G. (1994). Oxford House: Community living is community healing. *Addictions: Concepts and strategies for treatment.* (pp. 333-338). Gaithersburg, MD: Aspen.

Jason, L. A., Braciszewski, J. M., Olson, B. D., & Ferrari, J. R. (2005). Increasing the number of mutual help recovery homes for substance abusers: Effects of government policy and funding assistance. *Behavioral and Social Issues, 14,* 70-78.

Jason, L. A., Olson, B. D., Ferrari, J. R., & Davis, M. I. (2003-2004). Substance abuse: The need for second-order change. *International Journal of Self Help & Self Care, 2(2),* 91-109.

Jason, L. A., Davis, M. I., Ferrari, J. R., & Bishop, P. D. (2001). Oxford House: A review of research and implications for substance abuse recovery and community research. *Journal of Drug Education,* 31, 1-27.

Levy, J. M. (1995). *Essential Microeconomics for Public Policy Analysis.* Westport CT: Praeger Publishers.

McCrady, B. S., & Miller, W. R. (1993). *Research on Alcoholics Anonymous: Opportunities and alternatives.* New Brunswick, NJ: Rutgers University Press.

McLellan, A. T., Kusher, H., Metzger, D., Peters, R., Smith, I., Grissom, G. et al. (1993). The fifth edition of the Addiction Severity Index. *Journal of Substance Abuse Treatment, 9,* 199-213.

Molloy, P. (1993). *Self-run, self-supported houses for more effective recovery from alcohol and drug addiction.* Center for Substance Abuse Treatment: Technical Assistance Publication Series Number 5. U.S. Department of Health and Human Services. Rockwall, MD.

National Institute on Drug Abuse & National Institute on Alcohol Abuse and Alcoholism (NIDA). (1998). Chapter 1: Executive summary. In The economic cost of alcohol and drug abuse in the United States-1992. Retrieved January, 2002 from http//www.nida.nih.gov/economicCosts/Index.html

Nealon-Woods, M. A., Ferrari, J. R., & Jason, L. A. (1995). Twelve-step program use among Oxford House residents: Spirituality or social support in sobriety? *Journal of Substance Abuse, 7,* 311-318.

Olson, B. D., Jason, L. A., Ferrari, J. R., & Hutcheson, T. D. (in press). Bridging professional- and mutual-help: Applying the transtheoretical model to the mutual-help organization. *Journal of Applied and Preventative Psychology.*

Olson, B. D., Jason, L. A., Davis, M. I., Alvarez, J., & Ferrari, J. R. (2003). Community reintegration for formerly incarcerated offenders: The Oxford House model. Presentation of the American Psychological Association Convention, Toronto.

Ponitz, J. E., Olson, B. D., Jason, L. A., Davis, M. I., & Ferrari, J. R. (2006). Medical care of individuals residing in substance abuse recovery homes: An analysis of need and utilization. *Journal of Prevention & Intervention in the Community, 31* (1/2), 95-110.

Rajkumar, A.S., & French, M.T. (1997). Drug abuse, crime costs and the economic benefits of treatment. *Journal of Quantitative Criminology, 13*(3), 291-323.

Robert Wood Johnson Foundation. (1999). *Americans without health insurance: Myths and realities.* [Annual Report]. Princeton, NJ: Author.

Rosenthal, M. S. (1984). Therapeutic communities: A treatment alternative for many but not all. *Journal of Substance Treatment, 1,* 55-58.

Rosten, K. (2003). *Statistical Report for Fiscal Year 2002.* State of Colorado, Department of Corrections.

Salomé, H. J., French, M. T., Scott, C., Foss, M., & Dennis, M. (2003). Investigating variation in the costs and benefits of addiction treatment: Economic analysis of the Chicago Target Cities Project. *Evaluation and Program Planning, 26,* 325-338.

Schinka, J. A., Francis, E., Hughes, P., LaLone, L. & Flynn, C. (1998). Comparative Outcomes and Costs of Inpatient Care and Supportive Housing for Substance-Dependent Veterans. *Psychiatric Services, 49,* 946-950.

U.S. Department of Justice. (2003). *Cost-Benefits/Costs Avoided Reported by Drug Court Programs.* OJP Drug Court Clearinghouse, a program of the Bureau of Justice Assistance, Office of Justice Programs.

Yates, J. (1994). Toward the incorporation of costs, cost-effectiveness analysis, and cost benefit analysis into clinical research. *Journal of Consulting & Clinical Psychology, 62(4),* 729-736.

Zarkin, G. A., French, M. T., Mroz, T., & Bray, J. W. (1998). Alcohol use and wages: New results from the national household study survey on drug abuse. *Journal of Health Economics, 17 (1),* 57-71.

Zweben, A. & Fleming, M. F. (1999). Brief Interventions for Alcohol and Drug Problems. In Tucker, J. A., D. M. Donovan, & G. A. Marlatt (Eds.) *Changing Addiction Behavior: Bridging Clinical and Public Health Strategies.* Guilford Press: New York.

PART 3:
RESIDENTS IN RECOVERY

Chapter 7:
Stress and Coping:
The Roles of Ethnicity and Gender
in Substance Abuse Recovery

Justin T. Brown

City University of New York

Margaret I. Davis

Dickinson College

Leonard A. Jason
Joseph R. Ferrari

DePaul University

SUMMARY. This study investigated ethnic and gender differences in reported resource losses and gains for recovering substance abusers living in Oxford Houses (OH). Participants ($n = 829$) completed a version

---

Address correspondence to: Margaret I. Davis, PhD, Dickinson College, Department of Psychology, P.O. Box 1773, Carlisle, PA 17013-2896 (E-mail: davismar@dickinson.edu).

The authors received financial support from the National Institute on Drug Abuse (Grant # DA13231).

[Haworth co-indexing entry note]: "Chapter 7: Stress and Coping: The Roles of Ethnicity and Gender in Substance Abuse Recovery." Brown, Justin T. et al. Co-published simultaneously in *Journal of Prevention & Intervention in the Community* (The Haworth Press, Inc.) Vol. 31, No.1/2, 2006, pp. 75-84; and: *Creating Communities for Addiction Recovery: The Oxford House Model* (ed: Jason et al.) The Haworth Press, Inc., 2006, pp. 75-84. Single or multiple copies of this article are available for a fee from The Haworth Document Delivery Service [1-800-HAWORTH, 9:00 a.m. - 5:00 p.m. (EST). E-mail address: docdelivery@haworthpress.com].

of Hobfoll's (1998) Conservation of Resources (COR) Evaluation. Results indicated significant individual differences in resources, based on gender, ethnicity, and the length of OH residential stay. Men reported fewer resource gains and losses than women. With respect to ethnicity, African-Americans reported greater gains and losses in resources than European-Americans. Individuals with less time in an OH also reported having experienced more losses in the past three months. *[Article copies available for a fee from The Haworth Document Delivery Service: 1-800-HAWORTH. E-mail address: <docdelivery@haworthpress.com> Website: <http://www.HaworthPress.com> © 2006 by The Haworth Press, Inc. All rights reserved.]*

KEYWORDS. Oxford House, substance abuse, stress and coping

Hobfoll's (1988, 1998) *Conservation of Resources (COR) Theory* conceptualizes stress as a condition resulting from inadequate resources to effectively cope with life situations. COR theory uses economic terminology to quantify how people obtain, retain, and protect resources from potentially threatening situations (Hobfoll, 1998). According to COR, Regardless of how many resources one has in reserve, resource loss has a more significant (and detrimental) impact on a person than resource gain (Hobfoll, 2001). When resources are used to cope with stressors, they are depleted at a more rapid pace than when resources are used to obtain new or additional resources (Hobfoll, 2001). However, gains play a preventative role because they may be used at a later date to combat stress in midst of a crisis. Those people who begin with larger amounts of resources are less vulnerable to resource loss and are better equipped to gain further resources, which gives them a surplus of resources to rely upon during a loss spiral (Hobfoll, 2001).

Social support is an important resource individuals use to cope with stress. Cohen and Wills (1985) found that social support directly influences personal well-being and enables people to buffer against negative outcomes from highly stressful situations. Ethnic minorities traditionally rely on more informal forms of social support (e.g., family and friends) as opposed to more formal supports like social service agencies (Prelow & Guarnaccia, 1997). In addition, women compared to men are more likely to use social support networks to help cope with adversity (Hobfoll, 1986). Similar to ethnic minorities, women often have extra burdens related to having to deal with additional pressures from a society (e.g., often maintaining the home, childcare, and working a part-time or full-time job) (Hobfoll, 1986). These additional daily stressors place women under higher levels of strain.

Substance abuse is another factor that can influence the coping process. Some individuals may use psychoactive substances as a maladaptive way to cope with daily and chronic stressors (Ma & Henderson, 2002). Those individuals who initially use substances to relieve stress often later experience negative consequences and more stress associated with their use (Ma & Henderson). Similar to the downward spiral generally associated with resource loss, substance abuse often results in a spiral leading to a depletion of resources and deterioration of effective coping mechanisms (Davis, 2003). Additionally, Noone, Dua, and Markham (1999) found that individuals attempting recovery who had higher levels of stress had poorer sobriety levels because they frequently relied on substances to reduce stress.

The purpose of the present study was to examine the impact of ethnicity, gender, and substance abuse recovery on resources, losses and gains with individuals living in Oxford House (OH) recovery homes, which are self-governed, communal-living substance abuse recovery homes that involve no professional staff (see Jason, Davis, Ferrari, & Bishop, 2001). It was hypothesized in the present study that African-Americans, women, and individuals with less residential time in OH would report greater resource losses and fewer resource gains. Conceivably these individuals, lacking a substantial amount of initial resources, would have fewer resources available to cope with the substance abuse recovery process.

METHOD

Participants

Participants were current adult residents (*M* age = 38.75 years old, *SD* = 9.25) from one of over 170 national OHs who completed surveys as part of a larger National Institute on Drug Abuse (NIDA) funded study. Of the OH members surveyed, 92.5% (N = 829; 270 women, 559 men) were either African-American or European-American and reported histories of both alcohol and drug abuse. These poly-substance abusers were selected for the present study in order to control for possible discrepancies with single substance use. On average, participants reported they had completed 12.7 years (*SD* = 2.08) of formal education, had a previous monthly income of $1,210 (*SD* = $2,534), were sober from alcohol for 647 days (*SD* = 1,023 days) and from drugs for 656 days (*SD* = 1,010 days), and lived in an OH for 11 months (*SD* = 15 months).

Procedure

Participants were recruited through several methods. Research staff distributed flyers to all established Oxford Houses announcing the national study that was to be conducted by DePaul University. Three announcements were also published in monthly Oxford House newsletters. Recruiting was also conducted via letters to house presidents within selected geographic locations, followed by phone calls and house visits by research staff. In addition, individuals were recruited at an OH convention by the research team and asked to complete the survey onsite. In each case, research team members explained the nature, purpose, and goals of the accelerated longitudinal study. Then, staff reviewed the consent form, assured confidentiality, and all directions were read aloud throughout the survey administration. After completing the surveys, each participant received a $15 payment. Analyses were conducted to determine whether there were any important differences between participants based upon the method of recruitment and survey. Results of these analyses revealed no evidence that the different modes of recruitment and survey administration differentially influenced results of the study.

Six months was the median length of stay within an Oxford House. Those above and below this median were studied to assess if length of stay was related to the dependent variables. Previous research has shown that in substance abuse recovery, it often takes six months for stabilization to occur (Windle, Thatcher Shope, & Bukstein, 1996).

Measures

As part of a larger battery of measures, all participants in the present study completed the following demographic items: *age, gender, ethnicity, reported income from the previous 30 days, alcohol and drug sobriety*, as well as *length of time living in an Oxford House*. Participants also completed an abbreviated version of the *COR Evaluation* (Hobfoll, 1998), which had two sets of 45 items ("In the last 3 months, I have gained"; "In the last 3 months, I have lost") each with a 5-point Likert scale (0 = *not at all*, 1 = *a little*, 2 = *moderately*, 3 = *considerably*, 4 = *greatly*). Participants were first asked 45 items regarding *resource gains* followed by 45 items regarding *resource losses*. Each set of items summed to form two separate total scores for *resource losses* and *resource gains*, respectively.

RESULTS

No significant differences based on gender or ethnicity were found within the sample population regarding education, income, or sobriety from alcohol and drugs. Age was found to be significantly different between men and women, as well as between European-Americans and African-Americans. Therefore, in the analyses below, age was controlled for by using it as a covariate (however, adding this covariate did not change any of the study results).

A 2 (gender: women vs. men) by 2 (ethnicity: African-Americans vs. European-Americans) by 2 (length of stay in Oxford House: < 6 months vs. ≥ 6 months) *MANCOVA* was conducted, controlling for age, for the two dependent measures (*composite ratings* for *resource losses* and *resource gains*). Significant main effects for gender (Wilks' $\lambda = 0.97$, $F(1,805) = 11.69, p < .01$), ethnicity (Wilks' $\lambda = 0.94, F(1,805) = 26.57, p < .01$), and length of stay in OH (Wilks' $\lambda = 0.97, F(1,805) = 11.33, p < .01$) were found, as well as a significant interaction effect between gender and ethnicity (Wilks' $\lambda = 0.99, F(1,805) = 3.54, p < .05$).

Figure 1 displays the means for all groups based upon their reported COR losses and gains. For ethnicity, univariate analysis showed that African-Americans reported more significant gains ($M = 2.46, SD = 0.90$) than European-Americans ($M = 1.95, SD = 0.91$), $F(1,805) = 47.57, p < .01$, but there was no significant difference between African-Americans and European-Americans on resource losses. Univariate analysis also showed that men gained significantly fewer resources ($M = 2.07, SD = 0.96$) than women ($M = 2.29, SD = 0.88$), $F(1,805) = 8.77, p < .01$ and had significantly fewer overall losses of resources ($M = 0.87, SD = 0.79$) than women ($M = 1.03, SD = 0.83$), $F(1,805) = 8.02, p < .01$. Univariate analyses indicated a significant interaction effect between gender and ethnicity on the amount of resource loss, $F(1,805) = 7.07, p < .01$. African-American women reported the greatest amount of losses ($M = 1.12, SD = 0.97$) of all groups.

With respect to the length of stay in an Oxford House, individuals with less than 6 months of residence reported significantly more losses ($M = 1.07, SD = 0.86$) compared to individuals with 6 months or more residence ($M = 0.77, SD = 0.73$), $F(1,805) = 16.78, p < .01$.

FIGURE 1. Interaction Effects of COR Losses and Gains Between Ethnicity and Gender.

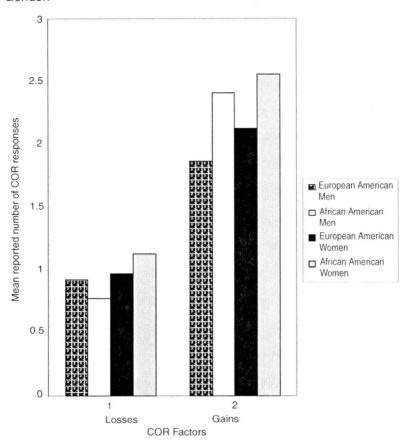

DISCUSSION

The present study found that ethnicity may impact coping for persons in substance abuse recovery. Historical implications suggest that African-Americans may have turned to alcohol as a way to escape from the stress of daily oppressive actions (Christmon, 1995). As a result, African-Americans may have learned maladaptive ways to cope with stress. Within the present study, African-Americans reported a significant amount of resource gains compared to European-Americans. This suggests that the supportive environment of an Oxford House may make a positive impact on the acquisition of coping resources for African-Americans recovering from substance abuse, and may positively impact the way they deal with stress associated with daily living and sobriety. According to Walton, Blow, and Booth (2003), African-Americans may have greater coping skills, but have more resource needs than European-Americans. The resource gains that African-Americans make in Oxford Houses are possibly because of having gained more stabilization within their lives, which allows them to work on replenishing and acquiring resources. The longer amount of time allowed by living in an Oxford House may allow African-Americans to end and reverse their loss cycles.

Regarding the main effect of gender, women may have more detrimental levels of resource loss in stressful situations than men. Hobfoll et al. (2003) found that stressful life events impact resources, and women with lower resource supplies tend to suffer greater loss if they have less effective coping styles such as inadequate social support networks, a reduced sense of self-mastery, and a sense of less control over their life. According to Boyd, Bland, Herman et al. (2002), women in recovery generally have more stressors, fewer positive life events, fewer coping resources, and more emotion-focused coping than other women. Women in recovery also may have children that they have lost custody of, or may be married to or dating another substance user (Dvorchak, Grams, Tate, & Jason, 1995). As a result, women in recovery suffer higher levels of unemployment and financial difficulties, legal issues, homelessness, and medical problems and poor physical health (Gehshan, 1993). The greater losses reported by the present sample of women in recovery from substance abuse may reflect this trend and suggests that women may have a continued spiral of experiencing losses after moving into there new living situation, thereby needing a longer adjustment period.

The importance of social support, especially to women in recovery, suggests that OHs may be an environment that is particularly helpful to them (Davis & Jason, 2004). In fact, Dvorchak et al. (1995) suggested that one of the primary benefits of an OH for women was offering a gender-specific environment that targeted their needs while in recovery. In addition, an OH setting may provide women a sense of personal empowerment by giving women the flexibility and autonomy to direct their own recovery program. The fact that in the present study the women also reported more resource gains than men, suggests that perhaps Oxford House creates a favorable environment for women to gain not only a positive social network, but also a place where women can acquire a variety of other important resources.

With respect to the interaction between gender and ethnicity, the finding that African-American men reported the least amount of losses while African-American women reported the most losses suggests that many of these women may come into Oxford Houses with limited resources to help them cope with sobriety. African-American women who abuse substances may have more difficulties because of their gender and ethnicity. According to Caetano and Clark (1998), African-American women typically have abstention rates higher than 55%, which is over 15% more than European-American women. Given this high abstinence rate, it is possible that those who do abuse substances have a great sense of guilt and greater negative consequences associated with their addiction history. African-American women in recovery may feel stigmatized within their culture because historically alcohol use has been discouraged by women within African-American communities (Christmon, 1995). This norm may cause African-American women greater reluctance in seeking treatment for their addictions, not seeking treatment until they have experienced significant losses. African-American women may also have a more difficult adjustment to the idea of treatment because of cultural factors as well as stress and historic experiences that influence their drinking patterns (Caetano, Clark, & Tam, 1998). Thus, African-American women may suffer from greater negative consequences and losses related to their use. Thus, perhaps these women would particularly benefit from an environment that halts the spiral of losses and encourages the gaining of resources such as Oxford House.

The present study also showed a main effect for length of stay indicating that individuals with less time in an Oxford House reported more resource losses. This finding was not surprising given that many important resources are typically depleted during regular substance use. However, Noone, Dua, and Markham (1999) found that persons recovering from alcohol abuse who had spent more time in substance abuse treatment had lower levels of stress and less inclination to relapse compared to other individuals in recovery. Therefore, it is likely that following entry into treatment, an adjustment period may occur within the first few months of recovery. Adjustments may include not only changes in previous use patterns but learning to cope within a new environment, social network, and possible employment opportunities. Within the context of Hobfoll's (1998) COR theory, some of the resources that are lost early in recovery transitions may be positive because the long-term effects may be more beneficial. Thus, although COR theory typically conceives of resource loss in negative terms, in the case of early substance abuse recovery, making important life transitions may involve a number of adverse losses but simultaneously include gains in effective resources. These resource losses (e.g., former networks of friend or communities that supported substance abuse) then may be considered "healthy losses."

The results of the present study suggest that it is important to explore the loss and gain of resources that may aid in coping with stress for persons in substance abuse recovery. The significant gender and ethnic differences in these processes also warrant further investigation. The present sample of participants were from Oxford House settings of individuals recovering from both alcohol and drug abuse. Oxford House residents may differ from other individual recovery because of the specificity of the Oxford House model. Also, all participants were questioned only about their previous 3 months of recovery. Some participants had been living in Oxford House during the prior 3-month time period while other participants had been living in another setting for part of this time. Along with this, participants' level of severity of substance abuse was not explored. These are several factors that may be worthy of consideration in future studies on these processes.

Though it appears Oxford House affects individuals' losses and gains of resources in different ways, the results of the present study showed that the Oxford House model may be beneficial to all residents, regardless of their ethnicity or gender. Furthermore, given a limitless length of stay policy, Oxford House may be an ideal recovery environment that allowed individuals sufficient time to stabilize their lives and reverse the trend through the gaining of valuable resources. Consistent with Oxford House's belief, the present study supported the notion that the substance abuse recovery process is individualized, varying for each person (OH Manual, 1988). However, over time, all participants seemed to benefit from living in an Oxford House because they were able to end the spiral of losses that may occur with substance abuse.

REFERENCES

Boyd, M. R., Bland, A., Herman, J., Mestler, L., Murr, L. et al. (2002). Stress and coping in rural women with alcohol and other drug disorders. *Archives of Psychiatric Nursing, 16*, 254-262.

Caetano, R., Clark, C. L., & Tam, T. (1998). Alcohol consumption among racial/ethnic minorities: Theory and research. *Alcohol Health & Research World, 22*, 233-238.

Christmon, K. (1995). Historical overview of alcohol in the African American community. *Journal of Black Studies, 25*, 318-330.

Cohen, S., & Wills, T. A. (1985). Stress, social support, and the buffering hypothesis. *Psychological Bulletin, 98*, 310-357.

Davis, M. I. (2003). Sex differences in alcoholics and addicts recovering in Oxford House: Exploring characteristics, social support, and self-efficacy (Doctoral dissertation, Depaul University, 2003). *Dissertation Abstracts International, 63*(12-B), 6089.

Dvorchak, P. A., Grams, G., Tate, L., & Jason, L. A. (1995). Pregnant and postpartum women in recovery: Barriers to treatment and the role of the Oxford House in the continuation of care. *Alcohol Treatment Quarterly, 13*, 97-107.

Gehshan, S. (1993). *A step toward recovery*. Washington, DC: Southern Regional Project on Infant Mortality.

Hobfoll, S. E. (1986). The ecology of stress and social support among women. In S.E. Hobfoll (Ed.), *Stress, social support, and women* (pp. 3-13). New York: Hemisphere.

Hobfoll, S. E. (1988). *The ecology of stress*. New York: Hemisphere.

Hobfoll, S. E. (1998). *Stress, culture, and community: The psychology and philosophy of stress*. New York: Plenum Press.

Hobfoll, S. E. (2001). The influence of culture, community, and the nested-self in the stress process: Advancing conservation of resources theory. *Applied Psychology: An International Review, 50*, 337-421.

Hobfoll, S. E., Johnson, R. J., Ennis, N., & Jackson, A. P. (2003). Resource loss, resource gain, and emotional outcomes among inner city women. *Journal of Personality and Social Psychology, 84*, 632-643.

Jason, L. A., Davis, M. I., Ferrari, J. R., & Bishop, P. D. (2001). Oxford House: A review of research and implications for substance abuse recovery and community research. *Journal of Drug Education, 31*, 1-23.

Ma, G. X., & Henderson, G. (2002). *Ethnicity and substance abuse: Prevention & intervention*. Springfield, IL: Charles C. Thomas Publisher, Ltd.

Noone, M., Dua, J., & Markham, R. (1999). Stress, cognitive factors, and coping resources as predictors of relapse in alcoholics. *Addictive Behaviors, 24*, 687-693.

Oxford House Manual. (1988). Silver Springs, MD: Oxford House, Inc.

Prelow, H. M., & Guarnaccia, C. A. (1997). Ethnic and racial differences in life stress among high school adolescents. *Journal of Counseling & Development, 75*, 442-450.

Walton, M. A., Blow, F. C., & Booth, B. M. (2001). Diversity in relapse prevention needs: Gender and race comparisons among substance abuse treatment patients. *American Journal of Drug & Alcohol Abuse, 27*, 225-240.

Windle, M., Thatcher Shope, J., & Bukstein, O. (1996). Alcohol use. In R. J. DiClemente, W. B. Hansen, & L. E. Ponton (Eds.), *Handbook of adolescent health risk behavior* (pp. 115-159). New York: Plenum Press.

Chapter 8:
Structural Social Support:
Impact on Adult Substance Use
and Recovery Attempts

Kerri L. Kim

University of Kansas

Margaret I. Davis

Dickinson College

Leonard A. Jason
Joseph R. Ferrari

DePaul University

SUMMARY. This study examined the structural social support of 132 men residing in a network of self-run, substance abuse recovery homes. The impact of different types of social relationships on individuals' substance use patterns and recovery attempts was investigated. Results sug-

Address correspondence to: Dr. Margaret Davis, Dickinson College, Department of Psychology, P.O. Box 1733, Carlisle, PA 17013-2896 (E-mail: davismar@dickinson. edu).

The authors received financial support from the National Institute on Drug Abuse (Grant # DA13231).

[Haworth co-indexing entry note]: "Chapter 8: Structural Social Support: Impact on Adult Substance Use and Recovery Attempts." Kim, Kerri L. et al. Co-published simultaneously in *Journal of Prevention & Intervention in the Community* (The Haworth Press, Inc.) Vol. 31, No.1/2, 2006, pp. 85-94; and: *Creating Communities for Addiction Recovery: The Oxford House Model* (ed: Jason et al.) The Haworth Press, Inc., 2006, pp. 85-94. Single or multiple copies of this article are available for a fee from The Haworth Document Delivery Service [1-800- HAWORTH, 9:00 a.m. - 5:00 p.m. (EST). E-mail address: docdelivery@haworthpress.com].

gest that varying relationship types (i.e., parents, significant other, friends, children, coworkers) have significantly different influences on use and recovery. Additionally, each type of relationship had differential impacts on use versus recovery. Children were the sole relationship type that affected both substance use and recovery attempts in a positive nature, suggesting that children may have a beneficial impact on reducing usage and prompting recovery in adults dealing with substance abuse issues. *[Article copies available for a fee from The Haworth Document Delivery Service: 1-800-HAWORTH. E-mail address: <docdelivery@haworthpress.com> Website: <http://www.HaworthPress.com>* © 2006 by The Haworth Press, Inc. *All rights reserved.]*

KEYWORDS. Social support, substance abuse, recovery

Studies have shown that general social support is related to an individual's overall physical and mental well-being (Burman & Margolin, 1992), while a lack of social support has been linked to the presence of problems such as substance abuse (McCrady, 1986). Findings have also suggested that while both general and abstinence-specific support contribute to better short-term drinking outcomes, the latter influences more long-term results (Beattie & Longabaugh, 1999). Moreover, Longabaugh, Wirtz, Zweben, and Stout (1998) found that involving individuals in a network of people who share a similar goal of maintaining abstinence may buffer them from the negative effects of a network that is supportive of substance use.

More recently, researchers have begun to examine the nature and characteristics of relationships that form an individual's support network. A recent meta-analytic review by Beattie (2001) supported that relationship function (i.e., content and purpose of interaction) and quality (i.e., subjective view of the relationship) are more predictive of drinking outcomes than relationship structure (i.e., the objective number and types of relationships that exist). However, no single result demonstrated more than a modest effect. While few studies have focused on relationship structure, Whisman, Sheldon, and Goering (2000) emphasized that the absence of close relatives was associated with alcohol abuse, while the absence of close friends was associated with several psychiatric disorders. In fact, being surrounded by even one supportive person may lead to better substance treatment outcomes, while being around just one person actively dealing with substance abuse issues may lead to more negative outcomes (McCrady, 2000).

Certain friendship qualities (such as trust, respect, usage status of the friend, and frequency of contact) have been associated with better outcomes among individuals in recovery (Humphreys, Mankowski, Moos, & Finney, 1999; Mohr, Averna, Kenny, & Del Boca, 2001). Relationships with family, which are generally long-term, also may contribute to the course of an individual's substance use and recovery attempts such that persons surrounded by family members emphasizing cohesion and expressiveness function better after treatment (Moos, Bromet, Tsu, & Moos, 1979). Being married to a person not dealing with substance abuse has also been shown to relate to more positive drinking outcomes (Beattie, 2001). In addition, the workplace is another environment that may facilitate the development of drinking norms and rationales (Rice, Longabaugh, & Stout, 1997). Finally, while the impact of several types of relationships (i.e., friends) on adult substance use and recovery attempts have been somewhat explored, the influence of children is an area that needs additional investigation.

Because substance abuse and addiction result from complex interactions between individual, social, and environmental factors (Fields, 1998), it is reasonable to speculate that effective treatment approaches will also utilize these interacting factors. Moreover, it suggests a need to further explore contextual, interpersonal, and individualistic variables, and to give due consideration to the dynamic processes that occur throughout recovery (Davis & Jason, 2004). Considering that substance abuse recovery homes address individual, social, and environmental issues, and are based upon the model of developing relationships of mutual help that encourage abstinence, they might be a particularly important setting to consider in the investigation of the impact of structural social support on the recovery process.

One such community-based recovery home program is *Oxford House*, where individuals deal with substance abuse recovery in a supportive, democratic, self-help setting with other persons in recovery (Ferrari, Jason, Olson, Davis, & Alvarez, 2003). Through living in the structured Oxford House environment, individuals develop and strengthen various important life skills which, in turn, may help recovering individuals maintain abstinence. Research on Oxford House (see Jason, Davis, Ferrari, & Bishop, 2001, for a review) suggests that it may be through fostering both social and individual resources that this innovative model promotes a process of recovery. Oxford House residents provide both general and abstinence social support for each other and actively encourage responsible, substance-free living. By residing in such an establishment, individuals' social support for abstinence and investment in those networks might increase, and this might positively impact individuals maintaining longer-term abstinence. Oxford House places residents in a context supportive of abstinence and removes them from the stressors, both situational and interpersonal, that may have been present in their previous communities. Furthermore, residents learn to develop and adjust their social network based on the need to surround themselves by individuals concerned with their recovery and overall well-being. However, little is known about the structural aspects of residents' social relations and their impact on use and recovery prior to and within Oxford House.

The present study examined the interpersonal relationships within individual social support networks of newer Oxford House residents–individuals living in an environment surrounding them with varying elements of the recovery process. Through this exploratory study, we investigated structural social support and assessed whether different relationship types (i.e., parents, significant others, friends, children, and coworkers) had an effect on use patterns and recovery attempts.

METHOD

Participants

Data used in this study was collected previously as part of a larger study of newly founded Illinois Oxford Houses for men. At the time of data collection, participants were current residents of 11 Illinois Oxford Houses and who had been living in an Oxford House for at least two weeks but no more than three months, with the average length of residence ranging between two to six weeks. The sample consisted of 133 male residents with a mean age of 33.8 years (range = 17-73). Thirty-five percent of the sample was African-American, 63% was European-American, and 2% represented other ethnicities, including Latinos. Most participants (55%) had never been married, 8% were presently married, and 37% had been married in the past (including those separated, divorced, and widowed). Of the sample, 17% earned a high school degree, 30% attained a high school diploma or GED, 42% had some college or vocational training, and 11% held a college degree or higher. A majority of individuals surveyed (64%) reported having current employment ($M =$ 754.85, $SD =$ 508.5). Lastly, 43.9% of the surveyed males reported having no children. Of those that did indicate having children, the mean number of children was 1.4 ($SD = 1.7$; range = 0-9).

Procedure

Participants were individually interviewed in a face-to-face manner by a trained volunteer research assistant. A second reliability observer was present at 50% of the interview sessions (inter-rater reliability = 90%). Brief 15-minute interviews were conducted on-site at the 11 Oxford Houses, located within and around Chicago, Illinois. After the initial greeting, the interviewer provided a description of the study and requested that the participant sign and date a consent form. Further, the interviewer highlighted that participation was voluntary and that the participant could choose to end the interview at any time. The survey used both closed and open-ended questions concerning participant choices and experiences with the recovery process.

Instrumentation

Participants were asked a number of sociodemographic questions (e.g., age, sex, education level, race, marital status, income, and number of children) as well as 19 questions regarding how and why the individual chose Oxford House as a treatment option, past issues (i.e., criminal, personal, medical), and previous recovery attempts. The two questions used in the present study addressed the individual's different social relationships and the impact of these relationships on substance use and recovery attempts. Participants were asked to rate how a variety of relationships (i.e., parents, significant other, friends, co-workers, and children) influenced their substance use and recovery attempts as having had either a *negative impact* (i.e., increased substance usage, decreased recovery attempts) *no effect*, or a *positive impact* (i.e., decreased substance usage, increased recovery attempts). The responses were coded as $-1 = negative\ effect$, $0 = no\ effect$, and $1 = positive\ effect$.

RESULTS

Differential Impact on Substance Use and Recovery Attempts

Initially we explored whether different types of relationships had varying effects on an individual's use and recovery (see Table 1 for means and standard deviations). General linear modeling was used to compare the types of relationships on their impact on substance use and substance abuse recovery. There was an overall significant effect for

TABLE 1. Means Scores for Impact of Relationship Types on Substance Use and Recovery–General Linear Model Comparisons (Within-Subject Repeated Measures)

	Parents	Significant Others	Children	Friends	Coworkers
Use[1]	−.15 (.47)[a]	−.31 (.58)[b,c]	.01 (.26)[a,b,d,e]	−.19 (.45)[d]	−.15 (.39)[c,e]
Recovery[2]	.21 (.45)[f,g]	.15 (.62)	.08 (.35)	.06 (.39)[f]	.05 (.27)[g]

$N = 120$
Note. Values in parentheses are standard deviations.
[1] For substance *use*, similar letters as superscripts indicate the means for relationship types are significantly different.
[2] For *recovery* attempts, similar letters as superscripts indicate the means for relationship types are significantly different.

different types of relationships, $F (4, 125) = 10.03$, $p < .01$. The Bonferroni correction was set at .005 for the subsequent planned comparisons. Five significant differences were found between relationship types. The influence of parents on use was significantly more negative from the influence of children, $F (4, 125) = 14.80, p < .005$. The impact of significant others on use was significantly more negative than the impact of children, $F (4, 125) = 37.94, p < .005$, and of coworkers, $F (4, 125) = 7.72, p < .005$. Finally, the effect of children on use was significantly more positive from the effect of friends, $F (4, 125) = 18.25, p < .005$, and coworkers, $F (4, 125) = 17.73, p < .005$.

For impact on recovery attempts, there was a significant overall effect between relationship groups, $F (4, 125) = 3.93, p < .001$ (see Table 1). Planned comparisons revealed that parental impact on recovery was significantly more positive than the impact of friends, $F (4, 118) = 10.51, p < .005$, and of coworkers, $F (4, 118) = 12.9), p < .005$.

Impact on Substance Use vs. Recovery Attempts

Additional analyses investigated the varying types of relationships and their differing affects on an individual's substance use versus recovery attempts. *Paired-sample t tests* were conducted with a Bonferroni correction (alpha criterion set at .01). Results suggest that for four of the five social relationships, the effect on substance use was significantly different from the effect on recovery. The perceived positive impact on recovery provided by parents, $t(128) = -6.26$, $p < .01$, significant others, $t(119) = -6.02$, $p < .01$, friends, $t(128) = -4.84$, $p < .01$, and coworkers, $t(128) = -4.70$, $p < .01$ was significantly greater than their negative impact on use patterns (see Table 1). Although the impact of children on participants' substance use and recovery attempts was not significantly different with the Bonferroni correction, children were the sole relationship type that presented a different pattern. Unlike the other four relationships, children impacted both use and recovery dimensions in a positive manner.

DISCUSSION

Results highlighted the overall influence of interpersonal relationships on substance use versus recovery attempts. Each relationship type impacted recovery in a positive manner, indicating that the important relationships in these men's lives were primarily endorsing the need for treatment and encouraging of recovery. Conversely, four of the relationship types (parents, significant others, friends, and coworkers) influenced use negatively, thereby supporting increased usage. The impact of children on substance use bordered on being a positive influence (see Table 1). Overall, these findings suggest a paradoxical role of interpersonal support. Given that relationships of individuals actively using substances are characterized by conflict (McCrady, 2002), it is reasonable to state that they serve as stressors and can contribute to the downward spiral of substance abuse. On the other hand, social relationships are complex, and enduring bonds may also serve as motivation to seek treatment and maintain substance abuse recovery.

Another important finding was that some relationship types (i.e., parents, significant others, and children) differed significantly on their impact on a person's substance use compared to one another, friends, and coworkers. Participants reported that all relationships (other than children) generally had a negative impact on their substance use. However, some relationships impacted individuals' substance use more than others. For instance, significant others displayed a more negative impact on use when compared to coworkers. It is reasonable to expect that coworkers would have less influence on an individual's use simply in part because of the capacity in which the relationship type functions. This notion addresses the need to encompass the overlapping structural, quality, and functioning elements of social support when discussing its impact on substance use and recovery. Participants also reported that all relationships were generally encouraging of their recovery attempts, and fewer significant differences were found when relationship type comparisons were conducted in regards to recovery. This highlights the importance of abstinence-specific support during the recovery process, irrelevant of relationship type (Zywiak, Longabaugh, & Wirtz, 2002).

Most interesting, children were the sole relationship type to impact use in a positive manner. While parents, significant others, friends, and coworkers presented with a pattern of negatively affecting substance use and positively affecting recovery, children were the only relationship type that presented as affecting both use and recovery positively. Although having children may contribute added concerns to the lives of adults using substances (e.g., dealing with child welfare services), current findings support the notion that children may provide motivation for recovery. Also possible is that since children were not living within the same residence as participants, the surveyed males were unable to attribute a more substantial impact to the role of children on their substance use or recovery. However, although we are able to speculate these explanations of results, the involvement of children in the substance abuse of their parents remains an issue largely unexplored (Arenas & Greif, 2000; d'Arlach, Curtis, Ferrari, Olson, & Jason, 2005).

The finding that significant others most negatively affect use compared to the other relationship types is also worth mentioning. In the most intimate of relationships, significant others can greatly influence the choices of their partners. McCrady (2002) reported that nearly 60% of surveyed individuals, who are dealing with alcohol related issues, report drinking with their partner. Therefore, if a significant other abuses substances, they are inherently providing their approval for increased usage. Additionally, active substance use adds a level of stress to interactions and so, continuing to use substances may be a coping strategy to lessen the immediate negative experiences.

In contrast to the impact of significant others on use, results demonstrate that parents have the most positive effect on recovery attempts. This finding suggests that the parent-child relationship, which is often thought of as relatively stable over the life span (Moos & Moos, 1984), may play a key function in supporting adult individuals throughout the recovery process and encouraging maintained abstinence. While recent research attempts have primarily focused on the role of parents in the substance abuse of adolescents (Henry, Robinson, & Wilson, 2003; Lochman & van den Steenhoven, 2002), our study suggests that parental impact may be an important factor in recovery throughout the life span. Given existing literature supports the importance of family involvement within the recovery process (Nakamura & Takano, 1991), more research is needed to investigate the influence of parents on adults dealing with substance abuse.

This exploratory study emphasized the key role support networks may have on substance abuse. However, the present study is limited in that no information was collected on women in recovery, thereby limiting generalization of structural social support for females. The qualitative-nature of the target questions may have allowed subjective interpretations of items, making it unclear whether participants referred to the same support network members for both substance use and recovery attempts. Clearly, future studies need to focus on comparing relationship types on their impact on substance use and recovery attempts. For instance, longitudinal data of structural social support paired with the maintenance of abstinence is needed and comparing Oxford House residents with individuals utilizing other treatment approaches should be conducted. Moreover, in trying to understand the different types of relationships, it is essential to clarify the beneficial role of children.

REFERENCES

Arenas, M. L., & Greif, G. L. (2000). Issues of fatherhood and recovery for VA substance abuse patients. *Journal of Psychoactive Drugs, 32*, 339-41.

Beattie, M. C. (2001). Meta-analysis of social relationships and posttreatment drinking outcomes: Comparison of relationship structure, function and quality. *Journal of Studies on Alcohol, 62*, 518-527.

Beattie, M. C., & Longabaugh, R. (1999). General and alcohol-specific social support following treatment. *Addictive Behaviors, 24*, 593-606.

Beattie, M., & Longabaugh, R. (1997). Interpersonal factors and posttreatment drinking and subjective well-being. *Addiction, 92*, 1507-1521.

Burman, B., & Margolin, G. (1992). Analysis of the association between marital relationships and health problems: An interactional perspective. *Psychological Bulletin, 112*, 39-63.

d'Arlach, L., Curtis, C., Ferrari, J. R., Olson, B. D., & Jason, L. A. (2005). Women, children, and substance abuse: A look at recovery in a communal setting. *Journal of Social Work Practice in the Addictions.*

Davis, M. I., & Jason, L. A. (2004). *Sex differences in social support and self-efficacy within a recovery community.* Manuscript submitted for publication.

Ferrari, J. R., Jason, L. A., Olson, B. D., Davis, M. I., & Alvarez, J. (2003). Sense of community among Oxford House residents recovering from substance abuse: Making a house a home. In A. T. Fisher, C. C. Sonn, & B. J. Bishop (Eds.), *Psychologi-*

cal Sense of Community–Research, Applications, and Implications (pp.109-122). New York: Kluwer Academic/Plenum Publishers.

Fields, R. (1998). *Drugs in perspective* (3rd edition). Boston, MA: McGraw Hill.

Henry, C. S., Robinson, L. C., & Wilson, S. M. (2003). Adolescent perceptions of their family system, parents' behavior, self-esteem, and family life satisfaction in relation to their substance use. *Journal of Child & Adolescent Substance Abuse, 13*, 29-59.

Humphreys, K., Mankowski, E. S., Moos, R. H., & Finney, J. W. (1999). Do enhanced friendship networks and active coping mediate the effect of self-help groups on substance abuse? *Annals of Behavioral Medicine, 21*, 54-60.

Jason, L. A., Davis, M. I., Ferrari, J. R., & Bishop, P. D. (2001). Oxford House: A review of research and implications for substance abuse recovery and community research. *Journal of Drug Education, 31*, 1-27.

Lochman, J. E., & van den Steenhoven, A. (2002). Family-based approaches to substance abuse prevention. *Journal of Primary Prevention, 23*, 49-114.

Longabaugh, R., Wirtz, P. W., Zweben, A., & Stout, R. (1998). Network support for drinking, Alcoholics Anonymous, and long-term matching effects. *Addiction, 93*, 1313-1333.

McCrady, B. (2002). *To have but one true friend: The role of families and others in recognizing and changing alcohol use disorders.* Presentation at the Annual Meeting of the American Psychological Association, Chicago, IL, August 2002.

McCrady, B. (1986). The family in the change process. In W. R. Miller & N. Heather (Eds.), *Treating addictive behaviors: Processes of change.* New York: Kluwer Academic Publishers.

Mohr, C. D., Averna, S., Kenny, D. A., & Del Boca, F. K. (2001). Getting by (or Getting High) with a little help from my friends: An examination of adult alcoholics' friendships. *Journal of Studies on Alcohol, 62*, 637-646.

Moos, R. H., & Moos, B. S. (1984). The process of recovery from alcoholism: III. Comparing functioning in families of alcoholics and matched control families. *Journal of Studies on Alcohol, 45*, 111-118.

Moos, R. H., Bromet, E., Tsu, V., & Moos, B. (1979). Family characteristics and the outcome of treatment for alcoholism. *Journal of Studies on Alcohol, 40*, 78-88.

Nakamura, K. & Takano, T. (1991). Family involvement for improving the abstinence rate in the rehabilitation process of female alcoholics. *The International Journal of Addictions, 26*(10), 1055-1064.

Rice, C., Longabaugh, R., & Stout, R. (1997). A comparison sample validation of "Your workplace": An instrument to measure perceived alcohol support and consequences from the work environment. *Addictive Behaviors, 22*, 711-722.

Whisman, M. A., Sheldon, C. T., & Goering, P. (2000). Psychiatric disorders and dissatisfaction with social relationships: Does type of relationship matter? *Journal of Abnormal Psychology, 109*, 803-808.

Zywiak, W. H., Longabaugh, R., & Wirtz, P. W. (2002). Decomposing the relationships between pretreatment social network characteristics and alcohol treatment outcome. *Journal of Studies on Alcohol, 63*, 114-122.

Chapter 9:
Medical Care of Individuals Residing in Substance Abuse Recovery Homes: An Analysis of Need and Utilization

Julie E. Ponitz

Wayne State University

Bradley D. Olson
Leonard A. Jason
Margaret I. Davis

Dickinson College

Joseph R. Ferrari

DePaul University

SUMMARY. The current study examined medical care need and utilization patterns among a substance abusing and recovering population

Address correspondence to: Julie E. Ponitz, Wayne State University, 71 West Warren Avenue, Detroit, MI 48202 (E-mail: jponitz@wayne.edu).

The authors appreciate the financial support from the National Institute on Drug Abuse (Grant # DA13231) and the National Institute on Alcohol Abuse and Alcoholism (Grant # AA12218).

[Haworth co-indexing entry note]: "Chapter 9: Medical Care of Individuals Residing in Substance Abuse Recovery Homes: An Analysis of Need and Utilization." Ponitz, Julie E. et al. Co-published simultaneously in *Journal of Prevention & Intervention in the Community* (The Haworth Press, Inc.) Vol. 31, No.1/2, 2006, pp. 95-110; and: *Creating Communities for Addiction Recovery: The Oxford House Model* (ed: Jason et al.) The Haworth Press, Inc., 2006, pp. 95-110. Single or multiple copies of this article are available for a fee from The Haworth Document Delivery Service [1-800-HAWORTH, 9:00 a.m. - 5:00 p.m. (EST). E-mail address: docdelivery@haworthpress.com].

(n = 876), investigating factors such as employment and drug use categories (e.g., pharmaceutical use, cocaine use, heroin use, alcohol use). It was found that those who were unemployed needed and utilized greater medical care than those who were employed. Results indicated that heroin, cocaine, and/or alcohol use was not predictive of medical care need or utilization, whereas pharmaceutical drug use was predictive of medical care need and utilization. Trauma and risky use of substances were not significant predictors of medical care need or utilization whereas the suicide severity composite was significant. Potential implications for misuse of medical services (e.g., to obtain pharmaceutical drugs of use) and federal medical care expenditure allocation are discussed. *[Article copies available for a fee from The Haworth Document Delivery Service: 1-800-HAWORTH. E-mail address: <docdelivery@haworthpress.com> Website: <http://www.HaworthPress.com> © 2006 by The Haworth Press, Inc. All rights reserved.]*

KEYWORDS. Medical care, addiction, Oxford House

Increasing medical care costs accrued by those addicted to drugs and alcohol indicate the importance of investigating predictors of medical need and utilization among this population. In 1995, over $34 billion was spent on medical costs associated with substance abuse not including treatment (Horgan, Skwara, Strickler, Andersen, & Stein, 2001). The general etiology and occurrence of illnesses and chronic health conditions associated with alcohol and drug abuse have been widely documented. Substance abuse has harmful effects on many organs including the liver, heart, pancreas, and nervous system (Rydberg & Skerfving, 1977), and users report more respiratory, cardiovascular, digestive, head/neck, eye, and general symptoms than nonusers (Patkar, Lundy, Leone, Weinstein, Gottheil, & Steinberg, 2002).

The abuse of illicit and legal (e.g., prescription) drugs and alcohol is commonly known to produce various cognitive deficiencies and, due to a greater tendency to engage in risk-taking behaviors, increase the risk for several infectious diseases including HIV (Scheidt, 1999). Additionally, alcohol and drug use can bring about and exacerbate the negative effects of malnutrition (Roggin, Iber, Kaber, & Tabon, 1969) and impair the function of the body's immune system, making addicted individuals more susceptible to bacterial and viral infections (Korsten & Wilson, 1999).

In addition to chronic illness and infection, severe and even terminal health conditions may arise from substance abuse. Individuals diagnosed with alcoholism are more likely to have the hepatitis-C virus (Rosman, Paronetto, Galvin, Williams, & Lieber, 1993), which may lead to cancer when the diagnosed individual does not cease their use of alcohol. Cancer, in general, has been strongly linked to alcohol consumption (Bognardi, Blangiardo, Vecchia, & Corrao, 2001; Longnecker, 1992). While the assertion that substance abuse directly incites health problems may be made, there are several uninvestigated factors other than chronic illness and infection that lead to medical care need and utilization. Characteristics and life-events of addicted and recovering populations may indicate what produces the greatest need for medical care and what increases the probability of utilizing such care.

One main cause for medical attention among substance abusing populations involves trauma and injury (Horgan et al., 2001). The probability of incurring injury and other health problems is impacted by risk taking behaviors, which are known to be elevated in those addicted to substances (Scheidt, 1999). An array of serious physical traumas such as traffic accident injury, criminal assault, accidental fall or burn, and accidental gunshot wound are commonly associated with substance abuse and its related risk-taking behaviors (Horgan et al., 2001; Subramanian, 2003). Treatment of these physical traumas tends to occur in hospital emergency room settings (SAMHSA, 2003; Horgan et al., 2001).

Related to physical injury and trauma among addicted individuals are suicide ideation and attempt, which are likely predictors of medical care need and utilization among this population. While little research has been conducted on suicide among this population (Farrell, Neeleman, Griffiths, & Strang, 1996), self-inflicted injury has been found to send a disproportionate number of individuals with substance abuse problems to the hospital (SAMHSA & OSP, 2003). Statistics show that the prevalence of suicide attempts among substance abusing populations is 5-7 times higher than the general population, with rates of 28% for males and 61% for females (Deykin & Buka, 1994). While those with substance-related disorders often suffer from depression and never see a physician or counselor, both suicide ideation and attempt directly result in more medical utilization (Deykin & Buka). Understanding the medical need and utilization of those whose physical and emotional states have reached a degree of severity in which they contemplate or concretely attempt to end their own life is essential in the struggle to provide care for those addicted to drugs and alcohol.

The particular substance a person abuses may also have a significant effect on their decision to obtain medical care, their need for medical care, and their subsequent utilization of services. In addition to the traditional drugs of use categories (such as alcohol, cocaine, and heroin), the abuse of prescription-type (i.e., pharmaceutical) drugs is becoming an increasing concern among addiction researchers and has a natural association with obtaining medical care (NSDUH, 2004; SAMHSA, 2003). Pharmaceutical drug abuse is defined as the non-medical use of drugs that have been designed with the purposes for treatment of medical conditions when appropriately prescribed by a physician (NSDUH, 2004). The pharmaceutical drug category includes sedatives, analgesics, tranquilizers/depressants, and barbiturates (NSDUH, 2004; SAMHSA, 2003; Simoni-Wastila, Ritter, & Strickler, 2004). Recent studies have shown that pharmaceutical drug abuse is rising in the United States, with the prevalence among the general population reaching rates equivalent to that of heroin and cocaine abuse (Goodwin & Hasin, 2002), and increasing among those addicted to traditional drugs use categories (Hesselbrock, Meyer, & Keener, 1985; Ross, 1993). Individuals who abuse pharmaceutical drugs may utilize more medical services when compared to those who do not, only to obtain the drugs to which they are addicted. Moreover, the utilization of services by those addicted to pharmaceuticals may be adding disproportionately to the annual federal expenditure on medical care compared to individuals who are not addicted to pharmaceuticals. Patterns of medical care need and utilization and drug use categories must be investigated among addicted and recovering individuals to understand medical service need and usage within this population.

Possibly of greatest importance in understanding medical care need and utilization is employment because it is often seen as an overarching predictor of substance abuse outcome and has many implications for medical care access and affordability (Robert Wood Johnson Foundation, 1999; Sindelar, 1991). Unemployed and/or uninsured individuals with substance abuse problems are often unable to pay for regular, maintenance medical care (RWJ, 1999). Costly emergency room services are frequently used by those addicted to substances and unemployed to obtain treatment for preventable illnesses and injury (RWJ, 1999). Given that emergency room visits cost over an average of $400 per visit (Horgan et al., 2001), the largely avoidable incidents and illnesses that result in addicted individuals' visits to emergency rooms are an ever increasing expense to society. Additionally, those who are uninsured or underinsured often experience delays in treatment, lack of treatment, and difficulty getting necessary medications (RWJ, 1999), often compounding already serious forms of illness or injuries and causing future treatment to be more expensive.

As research has shown, numerous health problems occur when individuals abuse alcohol and drugs and several factors influence the need that addicted individuals have for medical attention and their utilization of medical care. For instance, an addicted individual's employment status or specific drug of use may determine their access and reason for obtaining medical care. In an attempt to better understand the predictors of medical care need and medical care utilization by substance using and recovering populations, the current study investigated risk-taking behaviors, trauma, suicide ideation and attempts, drug use category, and employment as predictors of medical care need and medical care utilization. The current study hypothesized that greater risk-taking, recent trauma, greater suicidal ideation/attempts, and employment would be significant predictors of medical care need and utilization. Further, it was hypothesized that each drug use category and employment would predict medical care need and utilization.

METHODS

Participants

Participant information was collected at baseline from a larger National Institute on Drug Abuse (NIDA) funded national study of *Oxford Houses*, which are self-governing, communal-living aftercare environments that involve no professional staff (Jason, Ferrari, Smith, Marsh, Dvorchak, & Groessl et al., 1997). Analyses of records provided by Oxford House, Inc. using a geographical information systems program (Applegate, 1997), indicated that the majority of *Oxford Houses* across the United States generally clustered in five specific regions (Oxford House, Inc., personal communication, January, 10, 2002). These cluster areas included: Washington/Oregon, Texas, Illinois, Pennsylvania/New Jersey, and North Carolina. An accelerated longitudinal design was employed containing four waves of data, with each wave collected every four months (i.e., over the course of a year and a half). All participants were current residents of *Oxford Houses*.

The sample consisted of 896 residents (292 females, 604 males). The average age of the present sample was 39 (*SD* = 9.5, Range = 19.3-66 years) and was ethnically diverse: 58.5% European American, 34.1% African American, 3.5% Hispanic, 2% American Indian, and 2% other.

On average, education level reported by participants was 13 years and 77% reported being employed, while 23% reported being unemployed. Average monthly income was $1,005.00 ($SD = 2,487.00$). Consistent with the literature, suicide attempt and ideation was a prevalent occurrence in our sample with 46.6% of participants indicating they had experienced serious thoughts of suicide in their lifetimes and 30.1% participants indicated they attempted suicide in their lifetimes. Further, 11.6% indicated having had a plan to commit suicide and 7.3% had attempted suicide, in the last 12 months. Seventeen percent indicated they had experienced a physical injury or trauma, and 38% participated in risk-taking behaviors in the previous 12 months.

Procedure

Participants for the NIDA Oxford House study were recruited through two methods. The majority of participants ($n = 796$) were recruited by three announcements, published in monthly Oxford House newsletters distributed to all established *Oxford Houses*, which announced the national study and provided contact information. Recruiting was also conducted via letters to house presidents within the selected geographic locations, follow-up phone calls, and house visits by members of our research team. In addition, 100 individuals were recruited at the 2001 Oxford House World Convention.

In each case, the longitudinal nature, purpose, and goals of the study were explained to the participant. Staff members also explained that participation was entirely voluntary, participants were able to withdraw at anytime without pressure, and the consent form was reviewed in person with each participant. Preliminary analyses revealed no evidence that the different modes of recruitment and survey administration differentially influenced results of the study.

Survey Items

Among measures administered were the *Alcohol Severity Index,* the *Global Appraisal of Individual Needs at Intake-Quick,* and the *90-Day Time-Line Follow-Back.* Medical variables, medical care need and medical care utilization, were derived from the medical section of the *ASI* (McLellan et al., 1992; McLellan, Lubrorsky, Cacciola, & Griffith, 1985). Two medical care need variables, *how many days in the last 30 have you experienced medical problems,* and *how troubled or bothered were you by medical problems in the last 30 days* were derived from the

ASI. A single medical care utilization variable, *how many times in your lifetime have you been hospitalized*, was also derived from the *ASI*. One more medical care utilization variable was analyzed from the 90-Day Time-Line Follow-Back; *how many days in the last 90 were you hospitalized for medical problems*. The 90-Day Time-Line Follow-Back is a structured assessment interview for drinking and related behaviors developed by project MATCH (Miller, 1996; Tonigan, Miller, & Brown, 1997).

Drugs use category (pharmaceutical, alcohol, cocaine, and heroin) was analyzed from the *ASI* question, *have you used this substance for one or more years*. Employment status was derived from the ASI question, *on how many days in the last 30 have you been employed*. No composite scores from the *ASI* were calculated for the present study because our aim was to examine the specific information reflected by each item, not an overall pattern of severity. Also included in analyses were variables from the *GAIN-Q core*, a condensed version of the *Global Appraisal of Individual Needs-Intake*, intended to measure various life problems for adolescents and adults in various settings (Titus & Dennis, 2003). Variables incorporated from the *GAIN-Q core* included the suicide risk score, risky use of substances, and presence of trauma in the previous 12 months. The *GAIN-Q core* suicide risk measure is a composite score derived from five suicide action and ideation related questions with a Cronbach's alpha of .75 for adult populations (Titus & Dennis, 2003). Risky use of substances was determined from the questions: *during the past 12 months, have you kept using alcohol/drugs where it made the situation unsafe or dangerous for you, such as when you were driving a car, using a machine or where you might have been forced into sex or hurt*. Presence of trauma was determined from the question, *during the past 12 months, were you attacked with a weapon, beaten, sexually abused or emotionally abused*.

Analyses

Ordinary least-squares regressions were used to determine predictability of employment, suicide severity score, recent trauma, and risk-taking on medical care variables (i.e., *how many days in the last 30 have you experienced medical problems*, and *how troubled or bothered were you by medical problems in the last 30 days*) and medical care utilization variables (i.e., *how many times in your lifetime have you been hospitalized*, and *how many days in the last 90 were you hospitalized for medical problems*). To determine significant differences of medical care need and medical care utilization between drug use versus non-use, MANCOVA's were conducted with each drug of use category (i.e., pharmaceutical, alcohol, cocaine, and heroin) controlling for suicide severity score and ethnicity. Because employment has been found to be a central factor in utilization of medical services and substance abuse outcome (RWJ, 1999; Sindelar, 1991), it was included as a variable of primary interest in all analyses.

RESULTS

Descriptive Analysis

Preliminary descriptive analyses were conducted with all medical care need and medical care utilization dependant variables. Gender, ethnicity and level of education were tested and none were found to be significantly different with the exception of European Americans utilizing more lifetime medical services than African Americans, or any other ethnicity. Ethnicity, while an important variable, was not of specific interest in the current study and therefore controlled for in MANCOVA analyses.

Ordinary Least Squares Linear Regressions

Four ordinary least squares linear regressions were used to determine the relationships of each predictor on dependant variables, *medical care need* (i.e., how many days in the last 30 have you experienced medical problems, and how troubled or bothered were you by medical problems in the last 30 days) and *medical care utilization* (i.e., how many times in your lifetime have you been hospitalized, and how many days in the last 90 were you hospitalized for medical problems). Predictors in the model included *employment, suicide severity score, risky use of substances, and recent trauma.* Consistent predictors of the dependant medical variables were *employment* and *suicide severity score.* The effects for *employment* suggested that those who were employed had less lifetime hospitalization ($\beta = -.119$, SE =. 028, $p < .01$), less 90 day hospitalization ($\beta = -.146$, SE = .010, $p < .001$), had fewer days in which they had experienced medical problems in the last 30 days ($\beta = -.114$, SE = .027, $p < .01$), and were less bothered or troubled by current medical problems ($\beta = -.127$, SE = .005, $p < .001$) than individuals who were unemployed. With respect to *suicide severity scores*, those with higher, more severe suicide scores had moderately more lifetime hospitalization ($\beta = .607$, SE $= .324$, $p < .01$), more 90 day hospitalization ($\beta = .585$, SE $= .185$, $p < .01$), were more likely to have experienced medical problems in the past 30 days ($\beta = .894$, SE $= .444$, $p < .05$), and were more bothered or troubled by current medical problems ($\beta = .333$, SE $= .077$, $p < .001$). The independent variable *recent trauma*, was not a consistent predictor of the medical care variables, predicting one *medical care need* variable; how troubled or bothered an individual was by medical problems in the past 30 days, such that those who had experienced trauma in the last 12 months had more medical problems ($\beta = .524$, SE $= .158$, $p < 001$). Contrary to hypotheses, *risk taking* did not predict *medical care need* or *medical care utilization* variables.

Drug of Use Category Analysis[1]

Drug of use category was then examined with employment, in respect to the same four dependant variables: *medical care need* (i.e., how many days in the last 30 have you experienced medical problems, and how troubled or bothered were you by medical problems in the last 30 days) and *medical care utilization* (i.e., how many times in your lifetime have you been hospitalized, and how many days in the last 90 were you hospitalized for medical problems). Consistent with previous studies, drugs of a pharmaceutical origin (i.e., tranquilizers/sedatives, barbiturates, and analgesics) were collapsed into one drug use category (NSDUH, 2004; SAMHSA & OSP, 2003; Simoni-Wastila et al., 2004; Simoni-Wastila, 2000). Alcohol, cocaine, and heroin were also analyzed as drugs of use. MANCOVAs were conducted with each of the four drugs of use. *Suicide severity score*, the consistent significant predictor found in the regression analysis (other than employment), was controlled for in addition to ethnicity. Therefore, analyses were 2 (employment or no employment in the last 30 days) $\times$ 2 (drug of use addiction or no drug of use addiction) MANCOVAs.

Significant main effects held at the .01 level were found only with the pharmaceutical drug use category. Alcohol, cocaine, and heroin and their interactions with employment were not significant predictors of *medical care need* and *medical care utilization* variables. As Table 1 presents, omnibus test main effects were significant with pharmaceutical use, Wilks' λ (4,734) $= .961$, $p < .001$, employment, Wilks' λ (4,734) $=$

TABLE 1. Means and Standard Errors for Medical Care Need and Medical Care Utilization Variables as a Function of Lifetime Pharmaceutical Addiction and 30 Day Employment

	Lf Hosp.	90 Hosp.	Problems 30	Troubled 30
	M(SE)	M(SE)	M(SE)	M(SE)
Pharmaceutical Addiction				
Employed: 30 days	4.01(0.65)	0.26(0.20)	3.86(0.56)	1.00(0.20)
Unemployed: 30 days	9.80(1.22)	2.01(0.38)	6.75(1.06)	1.39(0.12)
No Pharmaceutical Addiction				
Employed: 30 days	2.70(0.52)	0.38(0.16)	2.50(0.45)	1.00(0.08)
Unemployed: 30 days	3.05(0.97)	0.79(0.30)	3.28(0.84)	0.94(0.16)

Note: Lf Hosp. = Number of times hospitalized in life
90 Hosp. = Number of times hospitalized in the last 90 days
Problems 30 = How many days have you had medical problems in the last 30 days
Troubled 30 = Degree of troubled or bothered by medical problems in the 30 days

.961, $p < .001$, and their interaction, Wilks' λ (4,734) = .979, $p < .01$. As displayed in Table 2, univariate results indicated pharmaceutical use was predictive of all *medical care need* and *medical care utilization* variables suggesting its strong influence on these factors. Univariate results on employment indicated it was a consistent predictor of *medical care utilization*, but was significant for only one *medical need variable*. This suggests that employment is closely linked with health care access issues and moderately related to need issues. Interaction effects between employment and pharmaceutical use were of greatest interest, and consistently predicted medical care utilization, but not medical care need. All means for the interaction effects between pharmaceutical use and employment status were in the direction such that those

TABLE 2. Multivariate and Univariate Analyses of Variance Wilks' and F ratios for Pharmaceutical Addiction X 30 Day Employment

	MANCOVA	ANOVA			
		Lf Hosp.	90 Hosp.	30 Problems	30 Troubled
	$\lambda(4,743)$	$F(1,751)$	$F(1,751)$	$F(1,751)$	$F(1,751)$
Pharmaceutical Addiction (P)	.961***	21.1***	4.40**	8.73*	3.86*
Employment: 30 Day (E)	.956***	13.1***	18.2***	7.70*	3.52
P × E	.979**	8.70**	7.48**	2.10	2.60
Suicide Severity	.974**	0.04	5.55*	6.76**	15.7***
European American	.999	0.36	0.00	0.21	0.01
African American	.997	0.03	0.71	0.93	0.06

Note: MANOVA = Multivariate Analysis of Variance; ANOVA = Univariate Analysis of Variance
Lf Hosp. = Number of times hospitalized in life
90 Hosp. = Number of times hospitalized in the last 90 days
Troubled 30 = Degree troubled or bothered by medical problems in the last 30 days
Problems 30 = How many days experienced medical problems in the last 30 days
Severity Score and Ethnicity were covariates
Ethnicity was recoded dichotomously. European American & African American were coded as *1* in each category; all 'other' ethnicities were coded as *0*.
***$p < .001$, **$p < .01$, *$p < .05$

with a pharmaceutical addiction and no employment tended to have more medical care utilization (refer to Table 1). These findings suggest that individuals addicted to pharmaceutical agents, especially those who are unemployed, are not more likely to have a need for medical care but are the most likely to utilize services among this addicted/recovering population.

DISCUSSION

One important finding of the study was that those addicted to pharmaceutical drugs had greater medical utilization, possibly suggesting that they may be accessing medical care more than others to obtain their drug of choice. Another consistent effect was that the strongest predictor of receiving medical attention was reflected in participants' suicidal inclinations. This finding, consistent with the literature, may indicate that those addicted to substances may not be receiving medical attention until their conditions are overly severe or until a situation occurs in which medical attention is unavoidable (e.g., being brought by an ambulance to an emergency room). Further, both sets of analyses indicated those who were unemployed needed and utilized more medical care. These results collectively reflect the discrepancies currently contributing to the immense, annual state and federal medical care expenditures due to substance abuse.

The finding that pharmaceutical drug use was a significant predictor of medical need and utilization, whereas use of alcohol, heroin, and cocaine were not, may contribute to a better understanding of the relationship between substance use and medical care if replicated in further studies. Those with a pharmaceutical addiction may objectively have more medical care need than those who are not addicted to this category of drugs. The pharmaceutical abuse of this group may have been initiated by an injury for which the individual originally obtained medication. However, subsequent long-term abuse of this drug category, as reflected in the current study, may involve obtaining further, unneeded medical care. The absence of findings for alcohol, heroin, and cocaine may suggest the use of these substances does not cause health issues. However, this is unlikely as these drug categories have been found to consistently cause serious and chronic health conditions that result in medical care utilization (Bognardi et al., 2001; Longnecker, 1992; Patkar et al., 2002; United States Secretary of Health and Human Services, 1993). Those addicted to pharmaceutical drugs may utilize more medical care due to *doctor shopping* (i.e., the practice of visiting several doctors to receive multiple, concurrent prescriptions to which an individual is addicted). This illegal method of obtaining drugs may expose these individuals to more medical settings which may familiarize them with medical conditions, thus increasing their ability to recognize health issues and report medical need.

Findings suggesting medical care may be most utilized by those with a pharmaceutical addiction have many policy implications. For instance, the results may indicate that money spent nationally on medical care for those who abuse substances may not be providing care for those most in need of medical treatment, but is instead lost on those addicted to pharmaceutical drugs who *doctor shop*. Furthermore, the unemployed among those addicted to pharmaceuticals utilized the most medical care, indicating they may be disproportionately incurring expenses when compared to employed drug users.

In all analyses, unemployment was found to significantly predict both greater medical care need and medical care utilization suggesting that those who are not employed may have a less stable, less healthy lifestyle. Although unemployment predicted more medical care need and utilization, it would be incorrect to assume that unemployed individuals have adequate access to medical care. Rather, unemployed individuals typically have less income and health care benefits which results in less access to health maintenance resources, such as voluntary check-ups and needed medications (RWJ, 1999). Because the uninsured are hospitalized more often for preventable illnesses, this may produce a substantially greater need, and subsequent utilization, of hospitalization in the unemployed versus the employed (RWJ, 1999). Therefore, greater utilization of medical care for the unemployed is likely a reflection of greater social and economic problems faced by this population. Costs accrued by unemployed, addicted persons receiving medical care, who are most likely uninsured and financially unaccountable for medical bills, are paid for by the premiums of the insured, and by federal and state taxes (Sindelar, 1991), and are thus a great cost to society. If more were invested nationally toward earlier treatment of medical and/or substance abuse problems, it is possible that this fiscal burden would be significantly lessened.

The possibility that addicted and recovering persons may often access health care only in cases of extreme severity is most reflected in the finding related to suicide. Suicide severity, like unemployment, was predictive of both medical care need and medical care utilization. Further indicating that those addicted to substances are not receiving timely care, were the findings that risk-taking did not predict either need or utilization and that trauma was only predictive of need. Throughout the substance abuse literature, these factors are found to create health problems, yet participants in the current sample did not utilize medical care when trauma or risk-taking occurred. One possible explanation for these results is that, despite all of the risk-taking behaviors and maladaptive health choices addicted individuals may make that should directly result in medical care, medical attention may only be given when it is involuntary (i.e., suicide-related hospitalizations). A congruent scenario is reflected in findings of past research showing that those addicted to drugs or alcohol tend not to be treated for medical problems until their situations are acute, either for compliance reasons, for fear of getting in legal trouble for use of illicit substances, or the tendency to numb pain/injury/affliction by self-medication (Khantzian, 1985).

Because of survey length limitations, specific medical history questions could not be included. Participants were not asked about routine medical care, such as check-ups and physicals, specific health issues, or specific reasons for hospital visits. In order to further understand the patterns of medical care need and utilization among addicted individuals found in the current study, additional research designed specifically to assess medical history and current and past health conditions is required. As the present study found consistent effects with employment status, issues such as access and availability to medical care should also be investigated among this population. Research has established the widespread negative health effects of addiction, billions of dollars are spent on the medical treatment for addicted populations each year, and yet treatment of the health problems commonly sustained by this population remains largely uninvestigated. Further understanding of such patterns may help researchers and practitioners better understand how to medically treat addicted individuals in need.

NOTE

1. To avoid poly-substance use confounding drug of use category analyses, correlations were performed between drug of use categories. No coefficient was strong enough ($r < .20$) to suggest confounding interactions.

REFERENCES

Anglin, M. K. & White, J. C. (1999). Poverty, health care, and problems of prescription medication: A case study. *Substance Use & Misuse, 34(14)*, 2073-2093.

Applegate, A. (1997). ArcView GIS (Version 3.2) [Computer software]. Redlands, CA: ESRI.

Bognardi, V., Blangiardo, C., La Vecchia, C., & Corrao, G. (2001). Alcohol consumption and the risk of cancer: A meta-analysis. *Alcohol Research & Health, 25(4)*, 263-270.

Deykin, E. Y., & Buka, S. L. (1994). Suicidal ideation and attempts among chemically dependant adolescents. *American Journal of Public Health, 4*, 634-639.

Farrell, M., Neeleman, J., Griffiths, P., & Strang, J. (1996). Suicide and overdose among opiate addicts. *Addiction, 91(3)*, 321-323.

Goodwin, R. D., & Hasin, D. S. (2002). Sedative use and misuse in the United States. *Addiction, 97(5)*, 555-562.

Hesselbrock, M. N., Meyer, R. E., & Keener, J.G. (1985). Psychopathology in hospitalized alcoholics. *Archives of General Psychiatry, 42,* 169-174.

Horgan, C., Skwara, K. C., Strickler, G., Andersen, L., & Stein, J. (Ed.). (2001). *Substance Abuse: The Nation's Number One Health Problem.* Princeton, NJ: Robert Wood Johnson Foundation.

Jason, L. A., Ferrari, J. R., Smith, B., Marsh, P., Dvorchak, P. A., & Groessl, E. J. (1997). An exploratory study of male recovering substance abusers living in a self-help, self-governed setting. *The Journal of Mental Health Administration, 24,* 332-339.

Khantzian, E. J. (1985). The self-medication hypothesis of addictive disorders: Focus on heroin and cocaine dependence. *American Journal of Psychiatry, 142,* 1259-1264.

Korsten, M. A. & Wilson, J. S. (1999). Health effects of alcohol. In R. T. Ammerman & P.J. Ott. (Eds.). *Prevention and societal impact of drug and alcohol abuse* (pp. 65-91).

Longnecker, M. P. (1992). Alcohol Consumption in Relation to Risk of Cancers of the Breast and Large Bowel. *Alcohol Health and Research World, 16(3),* 223.

McLellan, T., Kushner, H., Metzger, D., Peters, R., Smith, I., Grisson et al. (1992). The Fifth Edition of the Addiction Severity Index. *Journal of Substance Abuse Treatment, 9,* 199-213.

McLellan, T., Luborsky, L., Cacciola, J., & Griffith, J. (1985). New Data from the Addiction Severity Index: Reliability and validity in three centers. *Journal of Nervous and Mental Diseases, 173,* 412-423.

Miller, W. R. (1996). *FORM 90: A Structured Assessment Interview for Drinking and Related Behaviors, Test Manual.* Project MATCH Monograph Series, 4(Serial No. 96-4004).

National Survey on Drug Use and Health. (2004). *Non Medical Use of Prescription Pain Relievers.* Office of Applied Studies, Substance Abuse and Mental Health Services Administration. [Special Report]. Research Triangle Park, NC: RTI International.

Patkar, A. A., Lundy, A., Leone, F. T., Weinstein, S. P., Gottheil, E., & Steinberg, M. (2002). Tobacco and alcohol use and medical symptoms among cocaine dependent patients. *Substance Abuse, 23(2),* 105-114.

Robert Wood Johnson Foundation. (1999). *Americans Without Health Insurance: Myths and Realities. [Annual Report].* Princeton, NJ: Author.

Roggin, C. M., Iber, F. L., Kaber, R. M., & Tabon, F. (1969). Malabsorption in the chronic alcoholic. *Johns Hopkins Medical Journal, 125,* 321-330.

Rosman, A. S., Paronetto, F., Galvin, K., Williams, K. R., & Lieber, C. S. (1993). Hepatitis C Virus Antibody in Alcoholic Patients: Association with the Presence of Portal and/or Lobular Hepatitis. *Archives of Internal Medicine, 153(8),* 965.

Ross, H. E. (1993). Benzodiazepine use and anxiolytic abuse and dependence in treated alcoholics. *Addiction, 88,* 209-218.

Rydberg, U., & Skerfving, S. (1977). The toxicity of ethanol: A tentative risk evaluation, in Gross, M.M. (Ed.) *Alcohol Intoxication and Withdrawal: Advances in experimental medicine and biology* (pp. 403-419). New York: Plenum Press.

Scheidt, D. M. (1999). HIV risk behavior among alcoholic inpatients before and after treatment. *Addictive Behavior, Vol 24(5),* 725-730.

Simoni-Wastila, L., Ritter, G., & Strickler, G. (2004). Gender and Other Factors Associated with the Nonmedical Use of Abusable Prescription Drugs. *Substance Use & Misuse, 39(1),* 1-23.

Sindelar, J. L. (1991). Economics costs of illicit drugs: Commentary and Critique. In Economic Costs, Cost-Effectiveness, and Financing of Community Based Drug Treatment. *National Institute on Drug Abuse Research Monograph, 113*, 33-45.

Subramanian, R. (2003). *State Alcohol Related Fatality Rates 2002. Technical Report. December 2003.* Springfield, VA: Nation Highway Traffic Safety Administration. National Center for Statistics and Analysis: Advanced Research and Analysis.

Substance Abuse and Mental Health Services Administration, & Office of Sponsored Programs. (2003). *Emergency Department Trends from the Drug Abuse Warning Network, Final Estimate 1995-2002.* (DHHS Publication No. SMA 03-3780. Series D-24). Rockville, MD: U.S. Department of Health and Human Services.

Titus, J. C., & Dennis, M. L. (2003). *Global Appraisal of Individual Needs-Quick: Administration and Scoring Manual for the Gain-Q (version 2).* Bloomington, IL: Chestnut Health Systems.

Tonigan, J. S., Miller, W. R., & Brown, J. M. (1997). The reliability of Form 90: An instrument for assessing alcohol treatment outcome. *Journal of Studies on Alcohol, 58(4)*, 358-364.

Chapter 10:
African American Oxford House Residents: Sources of Abstinent Social Networks

Andrea M. Flynn
Josefina Alvarez
Leonard A. Jason
Bradley D. Olson
Joseph R. Ferrari

DePaul University

Margaret I. Davis

Dickinson College

SUMMARY. The current study found that African American residents of Oxford House (OH) used Narcotics Anonymous (NA) at high rates, and that both OH and NA strongly contributed to abstinent social networks. Having siblings and other family members in one's network predicted substance use among network members, whereas spouses, parents, and children did not have an effect on the rate of substance use.

Address correspondence to: Leonard Jason, Center for Community Research, DePaul University, 990 West Fullerton Avenue, Suite 3100, Chicago, IL 60614.

Funding for this manuscript was made possible by grants from the National Institute on Alcohol Abuse and Alcoholism (Grant #AA12218) and the National Institute on Drug Abuse (Grant #DA13231).

[Haworth co-indexing entry note]: "Chapter 10: African American Oxford House Residents: Sources of Abstinent Social Networks." Flynn, Andrea M. et al. Co-published simultaneously in *Journal of Prevention & Intervention in the Community* (The Haworth Press, Inc.) Vol. 31, No.1/2, 2006, pp. 111-119; and: *Creating Communities for Addiction Recovery: The Oxford House Model* (ed: Jason et al.) The Haworth Press, Inc., 2006, pp. 111-119. Single or multiple copies of this article are available for a fee from The Haworth Document Delivery Service [1-800-HAWORTH, 9:00 a.m. - 5:00 p.m. (EST). E-mail address: docdelivery@haworthpress.com].

These findings suggest that OH and NA may be effective sources of abstinent social support for African Americans recovering from substance abuse. However, family members are well represented in the support networks of African Americans in OH. *[Article copies available for a fee from The Haworth Document Delivery Service: 1-800-HAWORTH. E-mail address: <docdelivery@haworthpress.com> Website: <http://www.HaworthPress. com> © 2006 by The Haworth Press, Inc. All rights reserved.]*

KEYWORDS. African Americans, substance abuse, twelve-step programs, Oxford House

Several recent studies indicated that African Americans who abuse substances were significantly less likely than European-Americans to receive treatment (Liebman, Knezek, Coughey, & Hua, 1993; Wells, Klap, Koike, & Sherbourne, 2001). However, the 2000 National Household Survey on Drug Abuse revealed that 35.5% of African Americans over the age of 12 have used illicit drugs in their lifetime, as opposed to 41.5% of European Americans and 29.9% of Latinos (Substance Abuse and Mental Health Services Administration [SAMHSA], 2000).

Some research suggests that African Americans may use 12-step programs as a substitute for substance abuse treatment, whereas European-Americans use these programs in addition to professionally-led programs (Kaskutas, Weisner, Lee, & Humphreys, 1998). However, research on the utilization of 12-step groups by African Americans provides contradictory findings. In one study, Snowden and Lieberman (1994) found that, after controlling for use of professional services, 1.1% of the African American sample reported using self-help programs in their lifetime, compared to 3.6% of European-Americans. Similarly, Alcoholics Anonymous (AA) surveys indicate that African Americans receiving inpatient substance abuse treatment tend to under-utilize this self-help organization but are as likely to participate in outpatient treatment as European-Americans (Tonigan, Connors, & Miller, 1998). Humphreys, Mavis, and Stofflemayr (1991) found that African Americans leaving professional substance abuse treatment programs were more likely to attend AA than substance abusing peers that did not seek professional treatment, and such 12-step programs involvement contributes to greater length of sobriety for African-Americans (Roland & Kaskutas, 2002). Research has also indicated that African Americans are less likely to have a 12-step program sponsor than European Americans (Kaskutas et al., 1998). Together, these findings suggest that there is a need for more research exploring the experiences of African Americans in mutual-help organizations.

Social support is frequently identified as one of the main benefits of 12-step program involvement (Nealon-Woods, Ferrari, & Jason, 1995). For example, Toumbourou, Hamilton, U'Ren, Stevens-Jones, and Storey (2002) found that higher levels of investment and participation in Narcotics Anonymous (NA) predicted higher levels of social support. Humphreys and Noke (1997) examined the friend networks of males in substance abuse recovery and found that for individuals who utilized 12-step programs, involvement predicted both abstinent social support and number of friends. Involvement not only predicted a higher number of friends, but also increased frequency of contact with peers and overall quality of relationships (Humphreys & Noke). Kaskutas, Bond, and Humphreys (2002) found that social networks accounted for 36% of the effect of AA attendance among men and women in recovery from alcohol and drug use. Other research suggests that abstinent social networks are one of the most important predictors of substance abuse recovery following treatment (Longabaugh, Beattie, Noel, Stout, & Malloy, 1993; Zywiak, Longabough, & Wirtz, 2002). It is likely that support for abstinence may account for the effectiveness of 12-step programs in promoting abstinence.

The importance of family and friends in the social networks of African Americans has received much attention among social scientists (Prelow & Guarnaccia, 1997). However, Curtis-Boles and Jenkins-Monroe (2000) found that while non-substance abusing African American women indicated that their social support frequently came from family members, substance-abusing African American women were more likely to receive support from sources outside of the family, such as health professionals or 12-step program members. To date, however, little is known about the specific sources of social support and 12-step involvement as they may impact substance abuse recovery for African American men and women.

One mutual-help program that may provide a context to examine the role of social support in recovery is *Oxford House*. Oxford House may provide an affordable alternative to traditional modes of treatments for African Americans seeking recovering from substance abuse (Ferrari, Curtin-Davis, Dvorchak, & Jason, 1997). Previous research indicates that African Americans constitute nearly one-third of Oxford House residents (Bishop, Jason, Ferrari, & Huang, 1998) and African American men and women report that Oxford House positively contributes to their recovery (Ferrari et al.). Furthermore, Oxford House residents utilize 12-step groups (Nealon-Woods et al., 1995) while Oxford House itself may provide a mechanism for acquisition of abstinent social networks (Davis & Jason, 2004). However, little is known about the treatment history and specific recovery mechanisms for African American Oxford House residents (Ferrari et al., 1997). The present study examined the impact of 12-step program utilization and sources of social support for African American individuals living in Oxford House.

METHOD

Participants

A total of 305 African American residents were recruited to participate in a national study of Oxford House. Thirteen African American respondents were excluded because of insufficient information about their substance abuse histories, and 18 other respondents were excluded because they reported no previous illicit drug use. Of the remaining 274 participants, 181 (66.1%) were male, and 93 (33.9%) were female, ranging in age from 21 to 62 with a mean age in years of 40.8 ($SD = 7.4$). Many participants (47.4%) were single/never married, with a mean education level of 12.4 years ($SD = 2.27$) and most participants (70%) were employed full-time with an average monthly income of $1,081 ($SD = $2,563). The most common life-time substance reported as used by participants was alcohol, followed by cocaine, and cannabis.

Psychometric Measures

The Addiction Severity Index (ASI) (McLellan, Kushner, Metzger, Peters, Smith, Grissom, Pettinati et al., 1992) was used to provide recent and lifetime substance use along with medical, psychological, family, legal and employment problems as demographic information. The ASI composites, measuring 30-day alcohol and drug use, psychiatric, medical, employment and legal problems, are internally consistent (alphas $\geq$ 0.70) and demonstrate temporal stability (retest reliability $\geq$ 0.83; McLellan et al., 1992).

Alcoholic Anonymous Affiliation Scale (Humphreys, Kaskutas, & Weiner, 1998), a 9-item instrument, was used to assess the number of Alcoholics Anonymous and Narcotics Anonymous meetings participants attended in their lifetime and during the past 12 months. This scale also measures other aspects of participation in 12-step groups such as having a sponsor and reading literature, with scores ranging from 0 (*no twelve-step involvement*) to 9 (*high involvement*). The scale has good internal consistency (alpha = 0.85; Humphreys, Kaskutas, & Weisner, 1998). With the present sample, Cronbach's alpha was 0.85 for AA Affiliation and 0.79 for NA Affiliation.

The Important People Inventory (IP, Clifford & Longabaugh, 1991) asks participants to list up to 12 people that have been important to them and then to identify 4 of these individuals as the most important people. The measure is composed of 11 indices, including the following: number of people in the support network, the amount of contact with one's network, the average importance of the most important people, the substance use status of network members, the frequency with which network members use the network, the percentage of abstainers and recovering substance abusers in the network, the support for drinking among the most important people, and the average support for use among the most important people. The inventory's authors reported a coefficient alpha of 0.80 for the 11 indices combined (Longabaugh, Wirtz, Beattie, Noel, & Stout, 1995). Several subsequent studies, however, have reported lower alphas for the composite index and researchers have utilized various indices separately (Beattie & Longabaugh, 1999; Mohr, Averna, Kenny, & Del Boca, 2001). In the present study, the indices were weakly to moderately correlated, with a Cronbach alpha of 0.61 for the composite index. Consequently, we used percentage of abstainers in the social network and also included the percentage of Oxford House residents in participants' networks to explore the role of social support in Oxford House.

Procedure

Participants were recruited through letters to house presidents within geographic locations with high concentrations of Oxford Houses, followed by phone calls and house visits made by research staff. In addition, individuals were recruited at an Oxford House convention where research team members asked attendees to complete the survey onsite and by announcements in Oxford House newsletters.

In each case, research team members explained the nature, purpose, and goals of the study and read aloud all the measures. After completing the surveys, each participant received a $15 payment. Preliminary analyses revealed no significant differences in participant profiles or survey responses across the different modes of recruitment and survey administration.

RESULTS

Participants reported affiliation with NA (M = 6.44, SD = 2.11), AA (M = 4.58, SD = 3.31), and somewhat with Cocaine Anonymous (M = 1.32, SD = 2.12). To gain a better understanding of the impact of 12-step program affiliation on participants' social networks, *linear regression analyses* were conducted using the proportion of individuals in recovery as the dependent variable. Results (see Table 1) indicated that percentage of Oxford House members predicted the proportion of individuals in recovery in the social network. Additionally, even after controlling for percentage of Oxford House residents, NA affiliation remained a significant predictor of percentage of individuals in recovery in the social network. Length of time in Oxford House was not a significant predictor of the proportion of recovering individuals in participant's networks.

Participants' IP responses indicated that approximately 44% of their social support networks were composed of family members. On average parents accounted for 11% (SD = 17%), children 10% (SD = 20%), siblings 10% (SD = 16%), spouses 2% (SD = 6%), and other family members accounted for 11% (SD = 21%). Participants also reported a mean of 20% (SD = 26%) of their network as a 12-step friends or Oxford House residents. Boyfriends/girlfriends accounted, on average, for 7% (SD = 14%), ex-intimates for 2% (SD = 8%), coworkers for 2% (SD = 7%), and other friends for 11% (SD = 21%). *Linear regression analyses* also examined the proportion of family members as a predictor of heavy users in the network (see Table 2). Controlling for age, results indicated that the proportion of siblings and other family members in the network predicted heavy use among the participants' social networks, but this was not the case for the proportion of spouses, children or parents.

TABLE 1. Summary Regression Analysis for 12-Step Affiliation as a Predictor of Proportion of Recovering Members in Social Network

Variable	B	SE B	Beta
Proportion of OH members	.765	.067	.566***
NA Affiliation	.473	.163	.176**
AA Affiliation	−.062	.105	−.036
Length of stay in OH	.011	.023	.030

OH = Oxford House   **p < .01   ***p < .001

TABLE 2. Summary Regression Analysis for Percentage of Family and Age as a Predictor of Percentage of Heavy Users in Social Network

Variable	B	SE B	Beta
Proportion of spouses	−.180	1.04	.003
Proportion of children	.018	.331	.003
Proportion of parents	.147	.390	.024
Proportion of siblings	.797	.404	.123*
Proportion of other family	.657	.306	.132*
Age	−.007	.009	−.051

*$p < .05$

DISCUSSION

The results of the present study indicated that length of time in Oxford House was not significantly related to the proportion of Oxford House residents or individuals in recovery in the social network. This finding suggests that residents may start to receive the abstinent social support benefits of the Oxford House environment immediately. Additionally, results of the current study suggest that African American Oxford House residents use 12-step programs, consistent with previous studies of Oxford House residents (Nealon-Woods et al., 1995) but contrary to other findings. This study does not address the inconsistencies in the literature regarding 12-step utilization among African Americans. Thus it is possible that individuals who access Oxford House may be more likely to also utilize 12-step programs. An alternative explanation may be that Oxford House members encourage each other to participate in 12-step groups.

The results of the present study also revealed that having more Oxford House residents and involvement in NA predicted abstinent social networks for African American men and women. These findings suggest that NA and Oxford House may have separate but related contributions to recovering African Americans, extending the findings from Ferrari et al. (1997) and Nealon-Woods et al. (1995). Participants' social networks also included a higher proportion of family members than non-family members and only the proportion of siblings and other family members contributed to heavy use networks. Family members, therefore, seem to have an important effect on substance abuse recovery among African American Oxford House residents. Clearly, future research is needed to examine the quality and importance of relationships to African American Oxford House residents. Further attention also should be given to the specific relationship between family use and actual abstinence indicators, such as relapse.

REFERENCES

Beattie, M. C., & Longabaugh, R. (1999). General and alcohol-specific social support following treatment. *Addictive Behaviors, 24*, 593-606.

Bishop, P. D., Jason, L. A., Ferrari, J. A., & Huang, C. (1998). A survival analysis of communal-living, self-help, addiction recovery participants. *American Journal of Community Psychology, 26*, 803-821.

Clifford, P. R. & Longabough, R. (1991). *Manual for the administration of the Important People and Activities instrument: Project MATCH.* Unpublished document. Center for Alcohol and Addiction Studies, Providence, RI.

Curtis-Boles, H. & Jenkins-Monroe, V. (2000). Substance abuse in African American women. *Journal of Black Psychology, 26*, 450-469.

Davis, M. I. & Jason, L. A. (2004). *Sex differences in social support and self-efficacy within a recovery community.* Manuscript submitted for publication.

Ferrari, J. R., Curtin-Davis, M., Dvorchak, P., & Jason, L. A. (1997). Recovering from alcoholism in communal-living settings: Exploring the characteristics of African American men and women. *Journal of Substance Abuse, 9*, 77-87.

Humphreys, K., Kaskutas, L. A., & Weisner, C. (1998). The Alcoholics Anonymous affiliation scale: Development, reliability, and norms for diverse treated and untreated populations. *Alcoholism: Clinical and Experimental Research, 22*, 974-978.

Humphreys, K., Mavis, B., & Stofflemayr, B. (1991). Factors predicting attendance at self-help groups after substance abuse treatment: Preliminary findings. *Journal of Consulting and Clinical Psychology, 59*, 591-593.

Humphreys, K., & Noke, J. M. (1997). The influence of posttreatment mutual help group participation on the friendship networks of substance abuse patients. *American Journal of Community Psychology, 25*, 1-16.

Kaskutas, L. A., Bond, J., & Humphreys, K. (2002). Social networks as mediators of the effect of Alcoholics Anonymous. *Addiction, 97*, 891-900.

Kaskutas, L. A., Weisner, C., Lee, M., & Humphreys, K. (1998). Alcoholics Anonymous affiliation at treatment intake among White and Black Americans. *Journal of Studies on Alcohol, 60*, 810-816.

Liebman, J., Knezek, L. D., Coughey, K., & Hua, S. (1993). Injection drug users, drug treatment, and HIV risk behavior. In B. S. Brown & G. M. Beschner (Eds.), *Handbook on Risk of AIDS: Injection Drug Users and Sexual Partners* (pp. 355-373). Westport, CT: Greenwood Press.

Longabaugh, R., Beattie, M., Noel, N., Stout, R. L., & Malloy, P. (1993). The effects of social investment on treatment outcome. *Journal of Studies on Alcohol, 54,* 465-478.

Longabaugh, R., Wirtz, P., Beattie, M., Noel, N., & Stout, R. (1995). Matching treatment focus to patient social investment and support: 18-month follow-up results. *Journal of Consulting and Clinical Psychology, 63,* 296-307.

Longabaugh, R., Wirtz, P. W., Zweben, A., & Stout, R. L. (1998). Network support for drinking, Alcoholics Anonymous and long-term matching effects. *Addiction, 93,* 1313-1333.

McLellan, A. T., Kusher, H., Metzger, D., Peters, R., Smith, I., Grissom, G. et al. (1992). The fifth edition of the Addiction Severity Index. *Journal of Substance Abuse Treatment, 9,* 199-213.

Mohr, C. D., Averna, S., Kenny, D. A., & Del Boca, F. K. (2001). Getting by (or getting high) with a little help from my friends: An examination of adult alcoholics' friendships. *Journal of Studies on Alcohol, 62,* 637-645.

Nealon-Woods, M. A., Ferrari, J. R., & Jason, L.A. (1995). Twelve-step program use among Oxford House residents: Spirituality vs. social support in sobriety. *Journal of Substance Abuse, 7,* 311-318.

Prelow, H. M., & Guarnaccia, C. A. (1997). Ethnic and racial differences in life stress among high school adolescents. *Journal of Counseling & Development, 75,* 442-450.

Roland, E. J., & Kaskutas, L. A. (2002). Alcoholics Anonymous and church involvement as predictors of sobriety among three ethnic treatment populations. *Alcoholism Treatment Quarterly, 20,* 61-77.

Snowden, L. R. & Lieberman, M. A. (1994). African American participation in self-help groups. In T. J. Powell (Ed.), *Understanding the Self-Help Organization: Frameworks and Findings* (pp. 50-61).Thousand Oaks, CA: Sage Publications.

Substance Abuse and Mental Health Services Administration. (2000). *National Household Survey on Drug Abuse* (SAMHSA Publication No. 90-1681). Rockville, MD: Substance Abuse and Mental Health Services Administration. SAMHSA Office of Applied Studies: NHSDA Publications.

Tonigan, J. S., Connors, G. J., & Miller, W. R. (1998). Special populations in Alcoholics Anonymous. *Alcohol Health and Research World, 22,* 281-285.

Toumbourou, J. W., Hamilton, M., U'Ren, A., Stevens-Jones, P., & Storey, G. (2002). Narcotics Anonymous participation and changes in substance abuse social support. *Journal of Substance Abuse Treatment, 23,* 61-66.

Wells, K., Klap, R., Koike, A., & Sherbourne, C. (2001). Ethnic disparities in unmet need for alcoholism, drug abuse, and mental health care. *American Journal of Psychiatry, 158,* 2027-2032.

Zywiak, W. H., Longabough, R., & Wirtz, P. W. (2002). Decomposing the relationships between pre-treatment social network characteristics and alcohol treatment outcome. *Journal of Studies on Alcohol, 63,* 114-121.

Chapter 11:
Children, Women, and Substance Abuse:
A Look at Recovery in a Communal Setting

Lucía d'Arlach
Bradley D. Olson
Leonard A. Jason
Joseph R. Ferrari

DePaul University

SUMMARY. This study explored the sense of community among women ($n = 21$) and women with children ($n = 30$) living in Oxford Houses, with emphasis on how the presence of children might affect the household. Sense of community did not vary between participants with more or less than three months residence. Residents reported very high levels of satisfaction with the home, possibly because of a ceiling effect of little room for increases in their sense of community over time. Participants reported that they were getting along with the children in the home, that mothers could count on babysitting help, and that the children

---

Address correspondence to: Lucía d'Arlach, 2219 North Kenmore Avenue, DePaul University, Chicago, IL 60614 (E-mail: ldarlach@depaul.edu).

The authors would like to thank Kathy Erickson, Bertel Williams and Carmen E. Curtis for their contributions to data collection and this paper.

Funding for this manuscript was made possible by grants from the National Institute on Alcohol Abuse and Alcoholism (Grant # AA12218) and the National Institute on Drug Abuse (Grant # DA13231).

[Haworth co-indexing entry note]: "Chapter 11: Children, Women, and Substance Abuse: A Look at Recovery in a Communal Setting." d'Arlach, Luciá et al. Co-published simultaneously in *Journal of Prevention & Intervention in the Community* (The Haworth Press, Inc.) Vol. 31, No.1/2, 2006, pp. 121-131; and: *Creating Communities for Addiction Recovery: The Oxford House Model* (ed: Jason et al.) The Haworth Press, Inc., 2006, pp. 121-131. Single or multiple copies of this article are available for a fee from The Haworth Document Delivery Service [1-800-HAWORTH, 9:00 a.m. - 5:00 p.m. (EST). E-mail address: docdelivery@haworthpress.com].

had a positive effect on the household and their own recovery process. This effect did not differ between mothers and non-mothers, suggesting that non-mothers might view the children in the home with a sense of responsibility and sensitivity comparable to that of the mothers. Implications are discussed. *[Article copies available for a fee from The Haworth Document Delivery Service: 1-800-HAWORTH. E-mail address: <docdelivery@ haworthpress.com> Website: <http://www.HaworthPress.com>* © 2006 by The Haworth Press, Inc. All rights reserved.]

KEYWORDS. Women and mothers, Oxford House, sense of community

Between 1980 and 1995, few studies explored the parenting skills of addicted women (see Eliason & Skinstad, 1995). Moreover, studies linking poor child rearing to parental substance abuse relied on single case reports, retrospective information, or comparisons between the incidence of a given outcome between children of substance-abusers versus children of non-substance-abusers (Mayes, 1995). Thus, substance abuse alone may or may not be an indicator of dysfunctional parenting. Traumatic events for children–abuse, neglect and abandonment–are not limited to substance-abusing families (Mayes).

In the 1990s, a growing number of studies appeared showing that addicted mothers' entrance, retention and completion of treatment greatly increased when the threat of possible custody loss was removed and when custody arrangements were made for the child to reside with the maternal grandmother during the recovery process (DeLeon, 1997; Dvorchak et al., 1995; Hughes et al., 1995; Metsch et al., 1995; Szutser, Rich, Chung, & Bisconer, 1996). For example, Pajulo, Savonlahti, and Piha (1999) found that women were especially willing, and able, to reduce substance use during, and immediately after, pregnancy. The desire to stop abusing substances seemed predicated on a strong desire to be a good mother (Pajulo, Savonlahti, & Piha, 1999).

Paradoxically, treatment programs that include childcare facilities have high operating costs (Saunders, 1992), because state laws generally require 24-hour supervision of the children (Metsch et al., 1995). For example, *Project Together* that served 27 mothers and 31 children costs $665,000 annually (Metsch et al., 1995). Unfortunately, there are few recovery settings that address women's needs, and even fewer for women with children.

Oxford Houses are self-run recovery homes where six to eight individuals share a home and agree to remain abstinent, pay the rent, and avoid any disruptive behavior. Any violation of these rules leads to expulsion from the home (Jason, Ferrari, Groessl, & Dvorchak, 1997). Because Oxford Houses operate without professional staff, the residents cover the cost of their own recovery, and the low cost has allowed for the model to expand to over 1,000 Oxford Houses within the U.S. (Ferrari, Jason, Olson, Davis & Alvarez, 2002). Approximately 200 of these homes are for women, and 34 of them are for women and children (Ferrari et al., 2002). A small but growing body of research literature has been conducted on Oxford Houses (Ferrari et al., 2002; Jason, Ferrari, Dvorchak, Groessl & Molloy, 1997). Findings suggested that Oxford Houses offer women and women with children a setting where they can enhance their skills at long-term abstinence within a safe and supportive setting, and such a setting, in turn, assists mothers in the care of their children (Jason et al., 2002).

Self-help groups, such as Oxford Houses, may provide their members with a *psychological sense of community* (PSOC), a construct proposed by Sarason (1974) and refined by McMillan and Chavis (1986) and Bishop, Chertok and Jason (1997). Sense of community is the feeling of belonging to a mutually supportive network of similar others. This notion might be particularly important to substance-abusing women, who often have low social support (Harmer, Sanderson & Mertin, 1999) and feel intense shame over their addiction (Vanwesenbeeck, 1994). Social support is also vital in dealing effectively with the daily stresses of parenting (Harmer, Sanderson & Mertin, 1999).

The present study examined the interplay between sense of community, attitudes toward the presence of the children in the home, and parenting stress of mothers residing in an Oxford House. It was hypothesized that women's sense of community would increase over time in the Oxford House. Women's attitude towards the children's presence also would be directly related to their perceived sense of community, and that higher levels of sense of community would be associated with lower parenting stress levels felt by the mother. The role of ethnicity in on these variables also was explored.

METHOD

Participants. Participants were 51 women recovering from substance-abuse in an Oxford House for women and children. *Mothers* were defined as those women who had a biological child under the age of 18. Five women had children between the ages of 20 to 30 years old; therefore, these women were classified as non-mothers.

Procedure. Thirty-four Oxford Houses for women and children were identified and contacted by mail and phone. Two graduate students explained the purpose of the study over the phone to each house president while a written explanation and consent forms with stamped envelopes were mailed to each house. Approximately 25 women returned consent forms agreeing to participate. A second wave of phone calls and a packet of consent forms were mailed to each of the remaining houses, yielding a total of 51 participants (30 mothers, 21 women). All respondents agreed to be interviewed over the phone and mailed $15 compensation and insured of complete confidentiality.

Measures. A set of demographics questions (age, ethnicity, number of children, and Oxford House length of residency) selected from the *Addiction Severity Index-Composite (ASI-C:* McLellan et al., 1992) provided information about substance abuse, socioeconomic status, educational attainment, employment history, and legal status. The 30-item *Perceived Sense of Community Scale* (Bishop, Chertok, & Jason, 1997) measured women's sense of community experienced within the home. The scale's authors reported sufficient internal reliability (alpha = 0.95) for the entire scale. Also, participants completed the *Parenting Stress Index-Short Form (PSI-SF;* Abidin, 1990) assessing how mothers coped with the stress of parenting with at least one (youngest) child along three factors: *parental distress, parent-child dysfunctional interaction,* and *difficult child,* as well as providing an overall total score. Abidin (1995) reported the coefficient alpha was 0.91 for the total stress score, and > 0.80 for each of the factor scores; a score above 85 signified a high level of stress and above 90 a clinically significant level of stress.

Residents' attitudes toward children also were assessed with a 13-item, 5-point Likert scale created for this study called the *positive attitudes toward children questionnaire.* Sample items included: "I get along with the children in the house," and "The children's presence, whether your own or a housemate's, has a positive effect on my recovery." Cronbach's alpha was 0.84; therefore, we collapsed these items into a single score called the *Attitudes Toward Children* index. In addition, two 5-point Likert scale questions made up a *negative attitude toward parenting* questionnaire, namely: "I have complaints about the way some of the children's needs are met" and "I have complaints about the way some of the children in the house are disciplined." Cronbach's alpha was 0.88 for the two questions; therefore, we collapsed these two items into a single score.

RESULTS

Participant's Profile. Overall, the sample was composed of 47.1% European American, 47.1% African American, 4.6% Latina, and 1.2% Native American women. Mothers and non-mothers were similar in age, economic status, and legal history. Specifically, the average age of the women was 35.1 years old and the average number of years in school of each woman was 11.5 ($SD = 3.0$). On average, the women were employed 14.6 ($SD = 10.7$) of the last 30 working days and had 0.8 dependents to sustain financially ($SD = 1.0$). Women had been arrested and charged 10.1 times ($SD = 33.9$) and incarcerated a total of 7.8 months in their lifetime ($SD = 21.7$).

On average, participants engaged in 14.59 years of alcohol use ($SD = 9.9$), 3.07 years of heroin use ($SD = 6.2$), and 9.89 years of cocaine use ($SD = 8.9$). The sample had 2.16 ($SD = 2.1$) previous alcohol treatments and 3.28 ($SD = 3.2$) previous drug treatments. European Americans and African Americans reported similar substance abuse history, and no significant differences were found in the treatment history of both groups. Nevertheless, European Americans had slightly more previous alcohol treatments ($M = 2.38$, $SD = 2.2$) and drug treatments ($M = 3.42$, $SD = 4.1$) than African Americans ($M = 1.63$, $SD = 1.8$, and $M = 2.87$, $SD = 2.0$, respectively). While African Americans had fewer previous alcohol and drug treatments, they tended to stay in Oxford House two months longer on average ($M = 9.71$, $SD = 13.4$) than European Americans ($M = 7.29$, $SD = 7.9$), suggesting that the Oxford House model might be an effective treatment for African American women.

Children's Profile. In the present sample, 30 of the 51 women were mothers (i.e., women with children under the age of 18). Each mother had, on average, 2.3 children around 8.9 years old, yielding a total of 74 children under age 18. Approximately half of the 74 children (44.6%) had present or past involvement with the child protective services agency. At the time of the interview, most children were under the custody of their mother ($n = 43$, 58.1%) or relatives, especially grandparents ($n = 39$, 42.7%), while one resided with the father and one was in foster care. Finally, roughly half of the children ($n = 39$, 52%) had some contact with their fathers but not under his custody. Approximately half of the children had previous or current involvement with a child protective service agency ($n = 14$, 46.7%). Nineteen of the children were under the custody of their mothers (76.7%) and lived with her at the Oxford House.

Of the 11 children who did not reside with their mother, most tended to see their mother regularly. One mother saw her child daily while eight other mothers (26.7%) saw their child once or twice a week. Finally, two of the mothers saw their child infrequently, one on a monthly basis and the other, twice yearly. None of the child visits in this sample had to be supervised; all visits took place in the Oxford House, and usually lasted for the duration of a weekend. Only one visit had a time restriction limit of one to two hours.

Perceived Sense of Community

An *independent samples t-test* comparing women who resided in the Oxford House ≤ 3 months with women who resided in the house ≥ 3 months showed no significant differences in their self-report of perceived sense of community. Moreover, an *independent samples t-test* comparing the sense of community scores of mothers and non-mothers showed no significant difference, nor were any significant differences found between African American ($M = 122.43$; $SD = 14.30$) and European American ($M = 114.30$; $SD = 17.82$) women.

It was hypothesized that whether a resident was a mother or not and how a resident felt about the children and parenting in the house would affect their sense of community. *Multiple regression analyses* indicated that positive attitudes toward children was the only significant variable in predicting the perceived sense of community, $\beta = 1.05$, $SE = 0.29$, $p = .01$. In other words, a higher score on the attitudes toward children set of questions implied a more positive attitude toward the children's presence in the home. Negative attitudes toward parenting questionnaire, in contrast, did not significantly predict a sense of community, suggesting that residents ignore that negative parenting does not relate to sense of community.

Parental Stress

It was hypothesized that how frequently a mother saw her child, whether child protective services were involved in her life, and her perceived sense of community towards the home all would significantly predict parenting stress. An ordinary least squares regression was used to test the ability of frequency of contact with the child, child protective services involvement, and perceived sense of community to predict Parenting Stress Index scores (see Table 1). Only perceived sense of

TABLE 1. Means Scores on Parenting Stress Indices for African American and European American Women

	African American (n = 13)	European American (n = 15)
Parenting Stress Index:		
Parent distress	25.46 (3.7)	29.67 (6.2)
Difficult child	27.92 (5.8)	30.87 (6.0)
Parent-child dysfunctional interaction	23.23 (3.8)	24.33 (6.8)
Total score	76.62 (8.6)	84.87 (11.8)*

* $p < .05$
Note. Values in parentheses are standard deviation

community significantly predicted parenting stress by mothers, $\beta = -0.23$, $SE = 0.1$, $p = .04$. The mother's sense of community seemed to affect her parenting stress over other factors.

The Parenting Stress Index total score also was significantly different between African American and European American mothers, $t(26) = 2.37$, $p = .05$, with African Americans presenting a lower parenting stress mean than European Americans. When the subscales of the Parenting Stress Index were examined separately, the two groups only significantly differed in their scores on the *parental distress* subscale, $t(26) = 2.14$, $p = .04$, with African Americans presenting a lower average than European Americans.

DISCUSSION

The primary purpose of this study was to explore the sense of community within women and children's Oxford Houses, with a special interest on how the presence of children would affect the household.

Perceived sense of community did not vary in a cross-sectional comparison between residents who had been in the house more than three months and those who had been there less. One possible explanation for the results is that newly arrived residents reported great satisfaction with the home, creating a ceiling effect whereby a rise in the sense of community could not be captured. This was suggested by the high means, and is consistent with previous research where women, with or without children, reported having very positive expectations that their Oxford House would be a healthy environment with a strong fellowship (Ferrari et al., 2002).

Another interesting result was that the women's scores on the positive and negative attitudes toward children questionnaires predicted the sense of community in the household. The women reported that they were getting along with the children in the home, that the mothers could count on babysitting help, and that the children had a positive effect on the household and their own recovery process. This effect did not differ significantly between mothers and non-mothers, suggesting that women residents might view the children in the home with a sense of responsibility and sensitivity. Residents also were willing to help a fellow mother even if they disagreed with her parenting style. At the same time, residents seemed aware that poor parenting might disrupt the house.

These results suggest that children have a positive effect on every house member, not just the mothers. DeLeon (1997) and others (Hughes et al., 1995, Szutser et al., 1996) reported anecdotal evidence suggesting that children may provide a source of spiritual strength, serve to remind women of the negative effects of drug and alcohol use in the next generation, lower antisocial tendencies among women, as well as increase retention rates of mothers. In short, non-mothers may feel useful in contributing to the upbringing of the children, while mothers may find support from other women in the arduous task of parenting.

African American mothers reported significantly less parenting stress than European American mothers. Research indicated that African Americans compared to European Americans may be more likely to be punished for behavior associated with drug and alcohol use (McNeece & DiNitto, 1998) but less likely to receive substance abuse treatment (Mertens & Weisner, 2000). Taha-Cisse (1991) reported that minority women who abused drugs or alcohol while pregnant were 10-times more likely to be reported to child abuse authorities than European American women. Moreover, minority children have a higher incidence of foster placement because of parental drug use than European Americans (Jackson & Gordon, 1994). Because substance abuse may carry more serious consequences and treatment is more difficult to access for African American women, it is possible that the higher sense of community among African Americans was related to a higher motivation to succeed in treatment. Furthermore, African Americans may have felt more comfortable in a setting where trained staff were absent, alleviating feelings of distrust of authority. More simply, the communal setting environment of an Oxford House might be especially fitting to the African American culture; therefore, participants reflected a higher sense of community.

Implications for Women in Recovery

The present study offers several implications for the recovery process of women. For instance, in the present study, women's sense of community did not vary across time, implying that time alone may not improve or deteriorate a woman's process of recovery. A second implication of the present study was that self-help alone may not be enough for some especially complicated problems, such as mothers with clinically high parenting stress (Humphreys, 1997). A woman's Oxford House might want to screen for particularly high parenting stress levels and recommend a different setting or additional resources to such mothers, in order not to jeopardize the stability of the house. A third implication relates to the absence of a significant difference between mothers and non-mothers in their attitudes toward children. Treatment programs might consider mixing mothers and non-mothers within the same setting, to reduce the expensive costs of supervising and caring for a child's stay. Consequently, a woman's Oxford House might serve as a space for mothers seeking reunification to learn and practice parenting skills.

REFERENCES

Abidin, R. (1995). *Parenting Stress Index. Third Edition. Professional Manual.* Florida: Psychological Assessment Resources.
Abidin, R. (1990). *Parenting Stress Index. Short Form. Test Manual.* Virginia: University of Virginia.
Bishop, P. D., Chertok, F., & Jason, L. A. (1997). Measuring sense of community: Beyond local boundaries. *Journal of Primary Prevention, 18,* 193-212.
DeLeon, G. (Ed.) (1997). *Community as a method: Therapeutic communities for special populations and special settings.* Westport, CT: Praeger Publishers.

Dvorchak, P. A., Grams, G., Tate, L. & Jason, L. A. (1995). Pregnant and postpartum women in recovery: Barriers to treatment and the role of Oxford House in the continuation of care. *Alcoholism Treatment Quarterly, 13*, 97-107.

Eliason, M. J., & Skinstad, A. H. (1995). Drug/alcohol addictions and mothering. *Alcoholism Treatment Quarterly, 12*, 83-96.

Ferrari, J. R., Curtin, M., Dvorchak, P., & Jason, L. A. (1997). Recovering from alcoholism in communal-living settings: Exploring characteristics of African-American men and women. *Journal of Substance Abuse, 9*, 77-87.

Ferrari, J. R., Jason, L. A., Olson, B. D., Davis, M., & Alvarez, J. (2002). Sense of community among Oxford House residents recovering from substance abuse: Making a house a home. In A. Fischer, C. C. Sonn, & B. J. Bishop (Eds.). *Psychological sense of community: Research, applications, and implications.* (pp. 109-122). New York: Kluwer Academic-Plenum, Inc.

Harmer, A. L., Sanderson, J. & Mertin, P. (1999). Influence of negative childhood experiences on psychological functioning, social support, and parenting for mothers recovering from addiction. *Child Abuse and Neglect, 23*(5), 421-433.

Hughes, P. H., Coletti, S. D., Neri, R. L., Urmann, C. F., Stahl, S., Siciain, D. M. & Anthony, J. C. (1995). Retaining cocaine-abusing women in a therapeutic community: The effect of a child live-in program. *The American Journal of Public Health, 85*, 1149-1153.

Humphreys, K. (1997). Individual and social benefits of mutual aid self-help groups. *Social Policy, 27*, 12-19.

Jackson, M. R., & Gordon, L. B. (1994). Motherhood and drug-dependency: The attributes of full time versus part time responsibility for child care. *International Journal of Addictions, 29*, 1519-1535.

Jason, L. A., Ferrari, J. R., Groessl, E. J., & Dvorchak, P. A. (1997). The characteristics of alcoholics in self-help residential treatment settings: A multi-site study of Oxford House. *Alcoholism Treatment Quarterly, 15*, 53-63.

Mayes, L. C. (1995). *Substance abuse and parenting.* In M. H. Bornstein (Ed.), Handbook of Parenting, Volume 4. *Applied and Practical Parenting* (pp. 101-125). New Jersey: Lawrence Erlbaum Associates.

McLellan, A., Kushner, H., Metzger, D., Peters, R. et al. (1992). The fifth edition of the Addiction Severity Index. *Journal of Substance Abuse Treatment, 9*, 199-213.

McMillan, D.W., & Chavis, D.M. (1986). Sense of community: A definition and theory. *Journal of Community Psychology, 14*, 6–23.

McNeece, C. A. & DiNitto, D. M. (1998). *Chemical dependency: A systems approach.* Needham Height, MA: Allyn & Bacon.

Mertens, J. R. & Weisner, C. M. (2002). Predictors of substance abuse treatment retention among women and men in an HMO. *Alcoholism: Clinical & Experimental Research, 24*, 1525-1533.

Metsch, L. R., Rivers, J. E., Miller, M., & Bohs, R. (1995). Implementation of a family-centered treatment program for substance-abusing women and their children: Barriers and resolutions. *Journal of Psychoactive Drugs, 27*, 73-83.

Pajulo, M., Savonlahti, E., & Piha, J. (1999). Maternal substance abuse: Infant psychiatric interest: A review and a hypothetical model of interaction. *American Journal of Drug & Alcohol Abuse, 25*, 761-769.

Sarason, S. B. (1974). *The psychological sense of community: Prospects for a community psychology.* San Francisco: Jossey-Bass.

Saunders, E. (1992). Project together: Serving substance-dependent mothers and their children in Des Moines. *American Journal of Public Health, 82*(8), 1166-1167.

Szutser, R. R., Rich, L. L., Chung, A. & Bisconer, W.B. (1996). Treatment retention in women's residential chemical dependency treatment: The effect of admission with children. *Substance Use & Misuse,* 31, 1001-1003.

Taha-Cisse, A. H. (1991). Issues for African-American women. In Roth (Ed.), *Alcohol and drugs are women's issues. Volume One: A review of the issues* (pp. 54-60). Metuchen, NJ: Women's Action Alliance and Scarecrow Press.

Vanwesenbeeck, I. (1994). *Prostitutes' well-being and risk.* Amsterdam, Netherlands: VU University Press. 208 pp.

Chapter 12:
Women Leadership in Oxford House:
Examining Their Strengths and Challenges

Margaret I. Davis

Dickinson College

Marta M. Dziekan
Elizabeth V. Horin
Leonard A. Jason
Joseph R. Ferrari
Bradley D. Olson

DePaul University

SUMMARY. This study examined the perspectives and definition of leadership by women and mothers with children ($n = 40$) affiliated with Oxford Houses, a communal mutual-help recovery setting. Participants were asked questions relating to their experiences living in an Oxford House including the strengths and challenges encountered and how

Address correspondence to: Dr. Margaret I. Davis, Dickinson College, Department of Psychology, P.O. Box 1773, Carlisle, PA 17013-2896 (E-mail: davismar@dickinson.edu).

Gratitude is expressed to the women participants of the 2003 Oxford House Women's conference who participated in this survey study.

The authors received financial support from the National Institute on Drug Abuse (Grant # DA13231).

[Haworth co-indexing entry note]: "Chapter 12: Women Leadership in Oxford House: Examining Their Strengths and Challenges." Davis, Margaret I. et al. Co-published simultaneously in *Journal of Prevention & Intervention in the Community* (The Haworth Press, Inc.) Vol. 31, No.1/2, 2006, pp. 133-143; and: *Creating Communities for Addiction Recovery: The Oxford House Model* (ed: Jason et al.) The Haworth Press, Inc., 2006, pp. 133-143. Single or multiple copies of this article are available for a fee from The Haworth Document Delivery Service [1-800-HAWORTH, 9:00 a.m. - 5:00 p.m. (EST). E-mail address: docdelivery@ haworthpress. com].

doi:10.1300/J005v31n01_12

leadership impacted the stability in their house. Results illustrated the value of female leadership and highlighted the characteristics deemed important for women leaders in Oxford House, as well as some differences between these women's perception of leadership and the standard definition of leadership. The implications of the findings and how they may be useful to women's and mothers' with children houses are discussed. *[Article copies available for a fee from The Haworth Document Delivery Service: 1-800-HAWORTH. E-mail address: <docdelivery@haworthpress.com> Website: <http://www.HaworthPress.com> © 2006 by The Haworth Press, Inc. All rights reserved.]*

KEYWORDS. Leadership, women, Oxford House

In the United States, substance abuse has been typically identified as a male problem and thus treatment programs and models for treatment "have been designed primarily for males, culturally, demographically, and administratively" (Metsch, Rivers, Miller, Bohs, McCoy, Morrow et al., 1995). Furthermore, the overwhelming majority of substance abuse research has been conducted on men, with the results generalized to women, and most interventions–including prevention and treatment programs–have been based primarily on men's characteristics and needs (Leshner, 1998a). In addition, men designed and developed the majority of treatment programs (Abbot, 1994). These and other factors have contributed to a lack of conventional substance abuse programs which address the potentially different needs of women who have substance abuse problems (Davis & Jason, 2004).

The knowledge regarding women with drug/alcohol abuse and addiction that has accumulated thus far indicates these disorders may differ in etiology, have different consequences, and require different prevention and treatment approaches for women and men (Leshner, 1998b). Research on the origins of drug abuse found important sex-related differences in neurochemical and psychosocial factors affecting initiation, progression, and maintenance of drug use (Leshner, 1998b). NIDA-supported research also found significant sex-related differences in the medical, psychological, and social consequences of drug abuse (Leshner, 1998b). Additionally, research suggests that different psychosocial factors may influence women's and men's treatment progress and relapse to drug use following treatment (Leshner, 1998b). These findings together indicate a need to develop prevention and treatment programs that adequately address the unique needs of women and men in recovery.

It has been suggested that *Oxford House* (OH)–a national network of supportive, democratic, self-help settings, established and maintained by recovering alcoholics and addicts living together in order to develop long-term abstinence skills–may be an alternative to traditional treatment approaches that is suited to address the unique needs of women in recovery (see Davis & Jason, 2004; Dvorchak, Grams, Tate, & Jason, 1995). At present, of the greater than 1000 Oxford Houses (OHs) located in the United States, only 219 are homes for women and mothers with children (Oxford House, Inc., 2004). Among these female Houses are a number of well established and stable women's OHs that exemplify the potential of the OH model to support the recovery of substance-abusing women and mothers with children. Nevertheless, OHs for women and mothers with children have been reported to face many problems in terms of maintaining stability, and the factors that contribute to the instability of women's homes have been an area of concern and interest. One factor identified through conversations with alumnae of OH was an apparent lack of women in leadership positions. Anecdotal evidence suggests that even the highest functioning women's houses tend to have difficulties developing leadership within the house and consequently turn to more established and stable men's homes who may assume some of the women's leadership responsibilities.

Many studies suggest that women substance abusers also suffer from low self-esteem and poor self-concept. This also may impact the stability of the house and effect women's adoption of leadership roles (Marsh & Miller, 1985). However, it has been suggested that OH may be a recovery model in which the unique needs of women are met and important strengths and values are encouraged (d'Arlach, Curtis, Ferrari, Olson, & Jason, in press). Such things as increasing self-confidence, gaining knowledge and skills that are empowering are potentially related to both the OH model of recovery and leadership. According to Hensing, Spak, and Ostlund (2003), an atmosphere for women which nurtures leadership is one that prevents low-assertiveness and high emotionality, which are qualities that are often associated with alcohol dependence and drug use in women. However, to establish leadership in women, and women and children homes, the traditional conception of leadership may need to be altered. Because the traditional leadership structure within OH was designed under a male framework, this structure may not capture the different ideals and values that women associate with leadership. The present study explored these issues, specifically to gain a better understanding of leadership within women's OHs and how that role may relate to the stability of their homes.

METHOD

Participant Recruitment

On November 13, 2003, OH sponsored a one-day Women's Mini Conference in conjunction with the Oxford House (OH) World Conference in Washington D.C. The conference provided an opportunity for women involved with the OH community to come together and share and learn from each others' experiences. It was also an opportunity to investigate the experiences of women in OH and their feelings on leadership in these democratically-operated community-based recovery homes.

Survey Procedure

Data were collected from women who attended the Women's Mini Conference. In total, 60-70 women participated in some portion of that conference. The first author administered the survey at the conclusion of the mini-conference to the 40 women who attended the entire meeting. The survey took approximately 20 minutes to complete and included 34 closed and open-ended questions used for qualitative and quantitative analyses, respectively. Survey items addressed the following areas: content and format of the Women's Conference, leadership qualities that women deemed important, strengths and challenges of women's Oxford Houses and perceptions of the Oxford House experience in general.

Data Analysis Procedure

The quantitative data were analyzed using descriptive statistics to gather the frequency and percentages of each response. The qualitative data were coded based on the Grounded Theory approach (see Strauss & Corbin, 1998), in which open coding, axial coding and thematic coding methods were used as reference. During *open coding*, the data were coded without making any assumption about what was going to be uncovered. During *axial coding*, connections were made between categories and sub-categories in the data; and during *thematic coding*, data were grouped further into common themes that emerged. For each question asked, the answers were coded according to similarities and to determine themes. As an example of this method, all the answers that pertained to "personal characteristics" of individuals were grouped together and coded under that label. Within each group, answers were sub-grouped together according to further similarities. For example, "personal characteristics" related to personality traits were grouped together and differently from characteristics related to communication styles. The first and the second stages of coding occurred simultaneously. Through this process, common themes emerged for each question.

RESULTS

Of the 40 women who completed the study survey, 50% were alumnae and 50% were current residents of an Oxford House. Of these women, 55.9% lived in a women's house, while 29.4% lived in a women and children's house. The women represented numerous Houses across the nation. For instance, there were 12 women from North Carolina, 10 from Washington, four from Virginia, two each from Washington D.C., Kansas, and Illinois, and one each from Texas, Maryland, Oklahoma, Alabama, and Oregon. Of women attending the conference that filled out the survey, 82.9% considered themselves a leader in their house, while 17.1% did not consider themselves as leaders.

More than half of the women (65%) believed that effective leadership is an important factor that contributes to the success of a house; women reported on average a score of 4.8 (on a scale ranging from 1 = *not at all important* to 5 = *very important*) when asked to rate the importance of leadership in their OH (see Figure 1 for other factors that women felt were important to the success of their homes). Figure 2 depicts the characteristics that the women endorsed as being important leadership qualities of a woman in an OH. On qualitative items, respondents stated that good leaders in the house had knowledge of OH rules and were good role models without being overbearing or bossy. Additionally, these women felt that leaders were compassionate, open-minded, and listened to others making an effort to take action when conflicts arose. Finally, the women felt that good leaders were well established in the house (i.e., had spent a significant amount of time living there) and motivated others in recovery.

As well as exploring what leadership qualities women felt were a prerequisite to success in the women's OHs, respondents also answered questions regarding who the identified leaders in the house were. The OHs were run by a democratic process (80% majority rule) in which each house has a president and other service chairs and committee members. Elected terms for president varied, with some houses electing

FIGURE 1. The Percentage of Women Who Reported These Factors Determine the Success or Failure of a Women's House.

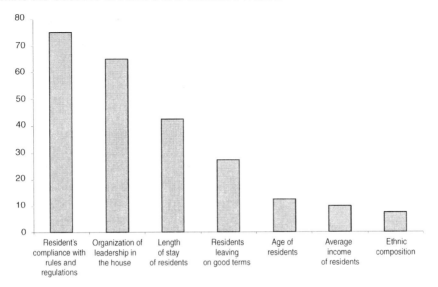

FIGURE 2. The Percentage of Women Who Indicated These Characteristics Are Important Leadership Qualities of a Woman in an OH.

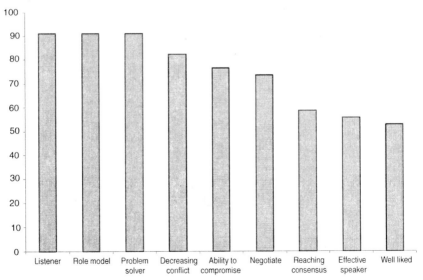

a new president every 6 months (91.4% of houses) and other houses electing a president every 3 months (2.9%) or less than every 3 months (5.7%). Results showed that while 25% of women saw the president as the identified leader in the house, 75% of women felt someone other than the president was the identified leader, with on average 2 persons per house perceived as leaders (range = 0-9). Furthermore, 68.4% of women believed that the president was not the most important leader in the house. These results suggest that women in OHs may conceive of leadership differently than a traditional model where one primary leader rules within a larger hierarchy. While the current president plays a leadership role in the house, other women (such as those who have been in the OH community for a long time, may also play an equally important leadership role).

Challenges to Leadership

Despite women's reporting of identified leadership within their own homes, 55.9% noted an insufficient number of women leaders within their Chapter. Also, when the house sought outside help to handle problems that arose, 34.4% of the women stated that the help came from men, 43.8% reported that they received help from other women, and 21.9% reported that they sought help from both women and men. The most commonly identified specific source that women turned to when they needed guidance was their local Chapter; specifically, the Chapter Chairperson. Additionally, six women reported that they sought out other OHs for guidance while six reported that others in the house sought them out. Five women sought help from the President of their own OH. Four people reported that they sought guidance from a state OH board representative, while four said they turned to each other. Lastly, three women noted that they sought guidance from housing service committee member(s) and three said they preferred help from senior members of the house. Two women also reported relying on an outreach organization (e.g., a Women's Outreach worker) for assistance.

DISCUSSION

Often women who enter an OH have had a series of negative life events such as histories of homelessness, trauma, and psychiatric co-morbidity, and little positive social support in their lives (Davis & Jason, 2004). Women in more traditional substance abuse treatments have also commonly been found to have considerable challenges and have more limited social support structures compared to men, with many of the relationships they possess being drug related (Marsh & Miller, 1985). However, in studies of women's treatment groups, women tend to perceive their peers as family (Marsh & Miller). To even greater extent, the communal living environment and the similar circumstances that bring the women of OH together may foster positive social support networks and the acquisition of important resources that can facilitate recovery (see Brown, Davis, Jason, & Ferrari, 2006). The current study supported the notion that the living environment of an OH may provide a space for women to build support networks that will aid them during recovery (Davis & Jason, 2004; Dvorchak et al., 1995). Half of the women reported on the survey that the bonding and harmony, as well as respect and mutual support were the greatest strengths of the women's houses.

The emphasis that these women put on mutual support as an aid to recovery, and their responses regarding leadership within their home suggests a conception of house leadership as a communal process rather than a hierarchical structure with one leader. The qualities that typified leadership in women's OHs were being a good role model, providing support and listening, good conflict resolution skills, and being dedicated to recovery. Although these qualities are in contrast to characteristics that are conventionally deemed important and necessary for a leader, such as aggression, competitiveness, dominance, ambition, and power (Klenke, 1996), they are in line with previous research on women leadership that has shown women leaders tend to highly value consideration and an interpersonal-orientation (DiMarco & Whitsitt, 1975; Petty & Bruning, 1980), and tend to adopt more democratic participatory leadership styles (Eagly & Johnson, 1990).

In contrast to traditional conceptions of leadership, which suggest one person has to rule over others (Klenke, 1996), women associated with OH feel that their house functions best when individuals both lead and follow. This is not to suggest that there are no leaders, but rather that simultaneously multiple women may serve as leaders. The majority of women in this study identified themselves as leaders and respondents indicated on average two leaders per house. However, it is important to note that the women attending this conference may have attended because they were identified as leaders in their community, suggesting these attendees were not representative of all female OH residents.

Nevertheless, 41.2% of participants reported that increased leadership would make a woman's OH run more smoothly and they desired more female leadership at the organizational, Chapter level. These opinions may partly be because there are more men's houses in a region that then dominate control, or, like other organizations, there are still relatively few women higher in the hierarchy within OH. Alternatively, these opinions may be partly attributable to the significant financial and time constraints placed on these women, particularly mothers with children, which makes it difficult to assume solo responsibility for a leadership role (Davis & Jason, 2004). Assuming a leader role may also be exceedingly taxing because of the multiple responsibilities and stressors these women face related to restructuring their lives during the course of recovery and concurrently also commonly dealing with other problems associated with prior negative and traumatic life experiences. Furthermore, taking on a leadership role early in recovery might seem challenging for many of the women in the OH given the low self-esteem that is typical for women with substance abuse problems.

In addition to the supportive environment that OH offers, both qualitative and quantitative data suggest that women's homes would benefit from more leadership in a non-traditional form and that this process of leading would benefit women's recovery. The multiple-leader structure endorsed by these women may offer alternatives to the traditional definitions of leadership. As noted, OH women report that they feel leadership involves working closely with other individuals and on a more intimate level. Providing more women within the house the opportunity to share leadership responsibilities could decrease the barriers to assuming such roles and also decrease some of the common problems that women mentioned leads to instability in the house. On the other hand, historically there have been some problems associated with more untraditional leadership models based on lack of structure and that such systems may increase the probability that individuals not take responsibility for their actions (Klenke, 1996). It has been noted that the women's movement in the 1960s lost considerable momentum when their intention to set up a system that would allow for participatory decision-making and shared responsibility, resulted in a system that lacked structure and was inefficient. Thus, women's houses may struggle with finding a balance between allowing many leaders and accomplishing goals, as was the case with the early women's grassroots movements. However, because a house is centralized, and the goal of sobriety is the same for all, there are likely to be fewer obstacles and greater benefits to adopting this organization over other more hierarchical structures.

This study suggests that considering alternate forms of leadership is important. Perhaps rethinking the conventional structure and characteristics of leaders might encourage more women to accept positions as leaders within the OH community. It is evident that women in OH believe that serving as a leader is an important role, and that OHs are stronger when there are effective women leaders involved with houses functioning. Furthermore, gender differences in leadership and differences in qualities and skills that women and men may value related to leadership should be further evaluated. Restructuring leadership positions so that they better fit the needs and capitalize upon the strengths of women may be essential to the ongoing success of OH.

Despite the many challenges faced by women in recovery, present survey indicated that OHs continue to be a positive community valued by women where they are able to make substantial changes in their lives. Anecdotal evidence suggested that there is great need for women to assume leadership positions within women's OHs and it seemed that these women felt that chapter- and state-levels are where female input as leaders was most lacking. Also, despite the common perception that women's houses are not as successful as men's houses, 63.3% reported that they feel women's houses were equally successful as men's OHs. Perhaps, women's houses may be perceived in a negative manner that is not entirely accurate. These findings speak to this issue and to the ability of OHs to offer an environment to women recovering from substance abuse that meets their needs and provides not only a supportive and safe atmosphere, but also one in which residents are able to become leaders in their home and community.

REFERENCES

Abbot, A. A. (1994). *A feminist approach to substance abuse treatment and service delivery.* New York: The Haworth Press, Inc.

Bond, M. A., Serrano-Garcia, I., & Swift, C. F. (2000). Women's empowerment: Review of community psychology's first 25 years. In J. Rappaport & E. Seidman (Eds.), *Handbook of Community Psychology* (pp. 857-886). New York: Kluwer/Plenum Publishers.

Brown, J. T., Davis, M. I., Jason, L. J., & Ferrari, J. R. (2006). Stress and coping: The roles of ethnicity and gender in substance abuse recovery. *Journal of Prevention & Intervention in the Community, 31*(1/2), 75-84.

d'Arlach, L, Curtis, C. E., Ferrari, J. R., Olson, B.D., & Jason, L. A. (2005). Substance-abuse women and their children: Cost-effective treatment options. *Journal of Social Work Practice in the Addictions.*

Davis, M. I., & Jason, L. A. (2004). *Sex differences in social support and self-efficacy within a recovery community.* Manuscript submitted for publication.

DiMarco, N., & Whitsitt, S. (1975). A comparison of female supervisors in business and government organizations. *Journal of Vocational Behavior, 6,* 189-196.

Dvorchak, P., Grams, G., Tate, L., & Jason, L. A. (1995). Pregnant and postpartum women in recovery: Barriers to treatment and the role of Oxford House in the continuation of care. *Alcoholism Treatment Quarterly 13,* 97-107.

Eagly, A., & Johnson, B. T. (1990). Gender and leadership style: A meta-analysis. *Psychological Bulletin, 108,* 233-256.

Hensing, G., Spak, F., Thundal, K. L., & Ostlund, A. (2003). Decreased risk of alcohol dependence and/or misuse is women with high self-assertiveness and leadership abilities. *Alcohol & Alcoholism, 38,* 232-238.

Hobfoll, S. (1985). *Stress, social support, and women.* Washington: Hemisphere Publishing Corporation.

Jason, L. A., Davis, M. I., Ferrari, J. R., & Bishop, P. D. (2001). Oxford House: A review of research and implications for substance abuse recovery and community research. *Journal of Drug Education, 31,* 1-27.

Klenke, K. (1996). *Women and leadership: A contextual perspective.* New York: Spring Publishing Company, Inc.

Marsh, J. C., & Miller, N. A. (1985). Female clients in substance abuse treatment. *The International Journal of the Addictions, 20,* 995-1019.

Metsch, L. R., Rivers, E. J, Miller, M., Bohs, R., McCoy, C. B., Morrow, C. J. et al. (1995). Implementation of a family-centered treatment program for substance-abusing women and their children: Barriers and resolution. *Journal of Psychoactive Drugs, 27,* 73-83.

McGraw, L. A., Zvonkovic, A. M., & Walker, A. J. (2000). Studying postmodern families: A feminist analysis of ethical tension in work and family research. *Journal of Marriage and the Family, 62,* 68-77.

Oxford House Manual. (1988). Silver Spring, MD: Oxford House, Inc.

Petty, M., & Bruning, N. (1980). A comparison of the relationships between subordinates' perceptions of supervisory behavior and measures of subordinates' job satisfaction for male and female leaders. *Academy of Management Journal, 23,* 717-725.

Saunders, E. J. (1993). A new model of residential care for substance-abusing women and their children. *Adult Residential Care Journal, 7,* 104-116.

Strauss, A., & Corbin, J. (1998). *Basics of qualitative research: Techniques and procedures for developing grounded theory.* Thousand Oaks: Sage Publications.

Index

BOOK ORDER FORM!

Order a copy of this book with this form or online at:
http://www.haworthpress.com/store/product.asp?sku=5613

Creating Communities for Addiction Recovery
The Oxford House Model

____ in softbound at $19.95 ISBN-13: 978-0-7890-2930-0 / ISBN-10: 0-7890-2930-8.
____ in hardbound at $39.95 ISBN-13: 978-0-7890-2929-4 / ISBN-10: 0-7890-2929-4.

COST OF BOOKS _____

POSTAGE & HANDLING _____
US: $4.00 for first book & $1.50
    for each additional book
Outside US: $5.00 for first book
& $2.00 for each additional book.

SUBTOTAL _____

In Canada: add 7% GST. _____

STATE TAX _____
CA, IL, IN, MN, NJ, NY, OH, PA & SD residents
please add appropriate local sales tax.

FINAL TOTAL _____
If paying in Canadian funds, convert
using the current exchange rate,
UNESCO coupons welcome.

❑ BILL ME LATER:
Bill-me option is good on US/Canada/
Mexico orders only; not good to jobbers,
wholesalers, or subscription agencies.

❑ Signature _____

❑ Payment Enclosed: $ _____

❑ PLEASE CHARGE TO MY CREDIT CARD:

❑ Visa ❑ MasterCard ❑ AmEx ❑ Discover
❑ Diner's Club ❑ Eurocard ❑ JCB

Account # _____

Exp Date _____

Signature _____
(Prices in US dollars and subject to change without notice.)

PLEASE PRINT ALL INFORMATION OR ATTACH YOUR BUSINESS CARD

Name

Address

City   State/Province   Zip/Postal Code

Country

Tel   Fax

E-Mail

May we use your e-mail address for confirmations and other types of information? ❑ Yes ❑ No We appreciate receiving
your e-mail address. Haworth would like to e-mail special discount offers to you, as a preferred customer.
We will never share, rent, or exchange your e-mail address. We regard such actions as an invasion of your privacy.

Order from your **local bookstore** or directly from
The Haworth Press, Inc. 10 Alice Street, Binghamton, New York 13904-1580 • USA
Call our toll-free number (1-800-429-6784) / Outside US/Canada: (607) 722-5857
Fax: 1-800-895-0582 / Outside US/Canada: (607) 771-0012
E-mail your order to us: orders@haworthpress.com

For orders outside US and Canada, you may wish to order through your local
sales representative, distributor, or bookseller.
For information, see http://haworthpress.com/distributors

(Discounts are available for individual orders in US and Canada only, not booksellers/distributors.)

Please photocopy this form for your personal use.
www.HaworthPress.com

BOF06